McGRAW-HILL PROBLEM SERIES IN GEOGRAPHY
Geographic Approaches to Current Problems:
the city, the environment, and regional development

Edward J. Taaffe, Series Editor

Wilfrid Bach
ATMOSPHERIC POLLUTION

Kevin R. Cox
CONFLICT, POWER, AND POLITICS
IN THE CITY: A Geographic View

Keith D. Harries
THE GEOGRAPHY OF CRIME AND JUSTICE

Richard L. Morrill and Ernest H. Wohlenberg
THE GEOGRAPHY OF POVERTY in the United States

Harold M. Rose
THE BLACK GHETTO: A Spatial Behavioral Perspective

Gary W. Shannon and G. E. Alan Dever
HEALTH CARE DELIVERY: Spatial Perspectives

David M. Smith
THE GEOGRAPHY OF SOCIAL WELL-BEING IN THE UNITED STATES:
An Introduction to Territorial Social Indicators

HEALTH CARE DELIVERY
SPATIAL PERSPECTIVES

GARY W. SHANNON
Assistant Professor of Geography
University of Florida

G. E. ALAN DEVER
Assistant Professor of Geography
Georgia State University

McGRAW-HILL BOOK COMPANY

New York St. Louis San Francisco Düsseldorf Johannesburg
Kuala Lumpur London Mexico Montreal New Delhi
Panama Paris Sao Paulo Singapore Sydney Tokyo Toronto

Library of Congress Cataloging in Publication Data

Shannon, Gary William.
Health care delivery: spatial perspectives.

(McGraw-Hill problems series in geography)
1. Medical care. 2. Medical geography.
3. Physicians. I. Dever, G. E. Alan, joint author.
II. Title
RA410.S5 610 73-11322
ISBN 0-07-056411-6
ISBN 0-07-05610-8 (pbk.)

Health Care Delivery: Spatial Perspectives

1 2 3 4 5 6 7 8 9 0 **KPKP** 7 9 8 7 6 5 4 3

This book was set in Baskerville by John T. Westlake Publishing Services. The editor was Janis Yates; the designer was John T. Westlake Publishing Services; and the production supervisor was Sally Ellyson

The printer and binder was Kingsport Press, Inc.

CONTENTS

EDITOR'S INTRODUCTION

From the middle of the nineteenth century to the present, studies have demonstrated the utility of the geographer's approach to problems of health and medical care. In the 1850s John Snow used a map of cholera cases to identify a contaminated well as the source of the epidemic, and Edward Jervis noted a consistent tendency for the per-capita use of mental hospitals to decline with distance. In *The Geography of Health Care,* Gary Shannon and G. E. Alan Dever present the results of a thorough survey of recent literature demonstrating the effects of distance and location on morbidity, frequency of consultation, referral practices, length of stay, and other aspects of medical care. In addition to map descriptions and interpretation, the authors make effective use of certain basic spatial models such as central place theory, distance-decay models, and variations of the gravity model in their analysis.

Professors Shannon and Dever examine the much-debated question of a physician shortage and come up with a convincing case for its existence, particularly in rural areas and poor, black neighborhoods. A damning example is that of two Chicago neighborhoods, one which has become predominantly black since 1930 and one which has remained predominantly white. The number of doctors in the black neighborhood declined from 122 to 44, while the number in the white neighborhood increased from 120 to 219.

In addition to providing students with a basis for identifying research problems, this book has a number of strong policy implications. The authors compare the system of medical care in the United States with those in the Soviet Union, Sweden, and England and conclude that Adam Smith's invisible hand is something of a blunt instrument when it comes to health planning. They present a scholarly, well-documented case for centralized and decentralized planning, as well as a more equitable delivery of medical services.

In this connection it is interesting to note that each of the other six volumes in the Problems Series, while not explicitly designed to be prescriptive, contains significant policy recommendations. *The Black Ghetto* stresses the need to recognize the cumulative nature of such hidden ghetto penalties as proximity of declining employment and noxious facilities. In *The Geography of Poverty,* the establishment of a guaranteed nonpoverty income is advocated. *Atmospheric Pollution* documents the inadequacy of existing air pollution laws. *Conflict Power and Politics in the City* emphasizes the need to reduce the increasing disparities between suburb and inner city in both tax bases and services. In *The Geography of Social Well-Being,* geographically disaggregated social indicators are called for. In *The Geography of Crime and Justice,* the author urges an end to the marked inequities in the administration of justice in different parts of the United States.

The Geography of Health Care is thus a welcome addition to the Problems Series. It is to be hoped that, in addition to stimulating broader research among geographers, it will cause some soul-searching among policy-makers charged with the regional planning of medical facilities and services.

Edward J. Taaffe

PREFACE

We are led to believe that apart from death and taxes nothing is more certain than change. Probably just as certain, however, is resistance to change. The present concern with the delivery of health care, particularly within the United States, results from an apparent overemphasis on progress and change in medical science and a failure or resistance to alter what must now be considered an outdated structure and inefficient organization relative to the deployment of health service delivery. Medical research and diagnostic procedures in the United States have achieved a sophistication almost without equal in the remainder of the world. Heart transplants, kidney transplants, effective immunizations, and cancer research programs are indicative of this high level of medical expertise. On the other hand, fundamental problems exist in the delivery of effective health care. Indeed, effective medical care, never readily available to lower socioeconomic groups, is apparently becoming increasingly remote from higher socioeconomic segments of the population. The United States, in 1973, is not yet committed to a comprehensive health care policy.

That the present "crisis" in medical care delivery should be the concern of a growing body of geographers suggests an added dimension to the traditional thrust of geographic investigation generally and medical geography in particular. Spatial perspectives of many of the problems currently endured by the United States as well as other countries, while certainly no panacea, are increasingly recognized as important to a better understanding of these problems and to any attempt to resolve them. In no area is geographic investigation and contribution more pertinent than in problems associated with the delivery of health services. In this context it is our hope that this book will be suggestive of a considered approach in the provision of medical care in an effective and efficient framework.

Certain geographic aspects of the health care problem are immediately recognizable. For example, the spatial patterns and variable distribution of health resources are basic issues to the delivery of effective medical care. Of course knowledge of the locational characteristics of medical resources and decision-making involved in a locational context by physicians are crucial to implementation of a successful mode of health care. Of special concern is the impact of geographic factors on the recipient, provider, and institutional policies. Such aspects as illness and therapeutic behavior, referral practices, and diffusion of innovative health care plans reflect areas that require a more systematic and comprehensive investigation. Finally, of particular interest is the spatial-functional organization of health care delivery of other countries. From these experiments, some more successful than others, we may derive information pertinent to the solution of our problem.

This work does not provide a remedy for the ills of America's health delivery system, rather it is a brief overview of geographic considerations of important facets which we feel must be included in any comprehensive approach to a solution of the problem. We hope this work suggests lines of inquiry and stimulates even greater concern on the part of health researchers to improved health care for the American people through the appropriate application of expanding expertise in spatial analysis.

CHAPTER I

HEALTH CARE DELIVERY: Introduction

An Overview

At the present time, the majority of observers agree that health care in the United States is experiencing a crisis. Among the manifestations of this crisis is an apparent decline in this country's rank among the developed nations of the world in its control of infant mortality, maladies associated with old age, and death from various diseases. This decline, plus the continuing rapid increase in the cost of health care, have given rise to a general uneasiness among the population. This uneasy populace may be best described by a statement attributed to Herman Hickman regarding the Yale alumni during a losing football season as being "surly but not rebellious."

Some of the underlying problems that have been identified by observers include the following: (1) an inadequate health insurance scheme; (2) a shortage of physicians and a maldistribution of existing physicians; (3) differential accessibility to health services; (4) differential availability of health services for various segments of the population; and (5) lack of coordination of health and city and regional planning. These problems are occurring in the country that has become the world's first service economy—the first country in which more than half of the employed population produces services instead of tangible goods. [1]

Emotions related to the above problems are apparently so general and pervasive that it is no longer useful to assign blame or responsibility either to the private or the public sector. It is useful, however, to examine selected facets of the complex health care problems and to demonstrate their geographical or spatial components. This type of investigation will provide a better understanding of the health care process and subsequent improved planning for health delivery systems. For this reason, the major purpose of this effort is to extend and supplement the more traditional concepts of medical geography, many of which have been preempted by the medical profession.[2]

Medical Geography – Traditional Considerations

An illustrative example of the traditional relationship between geography and medicine is provided by L. L. Finke, a German clinician, who wrote in 1792:

> When one deals with country after country, and with regard to each describes its position, the conditions of its soil, the peculiarities of the air, the water, the weather, and the foodstuffs used by the natives; when one describes the modes of life, customs and habits of the people insofar as they have anything to do with health and disease; when one gives account of the diseases themselves as found in different countries, and the local therapeutic measures; in short, when one brings together all which is worth knowing with regard to the medical status of any country then no one can deny that such a work deserves the name medical geography."[3]

On a more practical level medical geography or geographic pathology has implied comparative studies among different ethnic, national, or social groups. These studies generally correlate features of the social and geographical environments to data on the incidence of disease and the distribution of physiological traits in people belonging to different communities throughout the world.[4]

Whether this area of interest be denoted as medical geography or geographic pathology, the contributions are many. The classic example of a medical geography study is by Dr. John Snow, a general practitioner in the Gold Square area of London, who observed a causal link between cholera and water. In one section of London in 1854, over five hundred cholera deaths occurred within ten days. Dr. Snow, proceeded to plot on a large scale map

(Figure 1.1) the exact residence of each victim. Through visual analysis of the cholera distribution, he discovered that the deaths

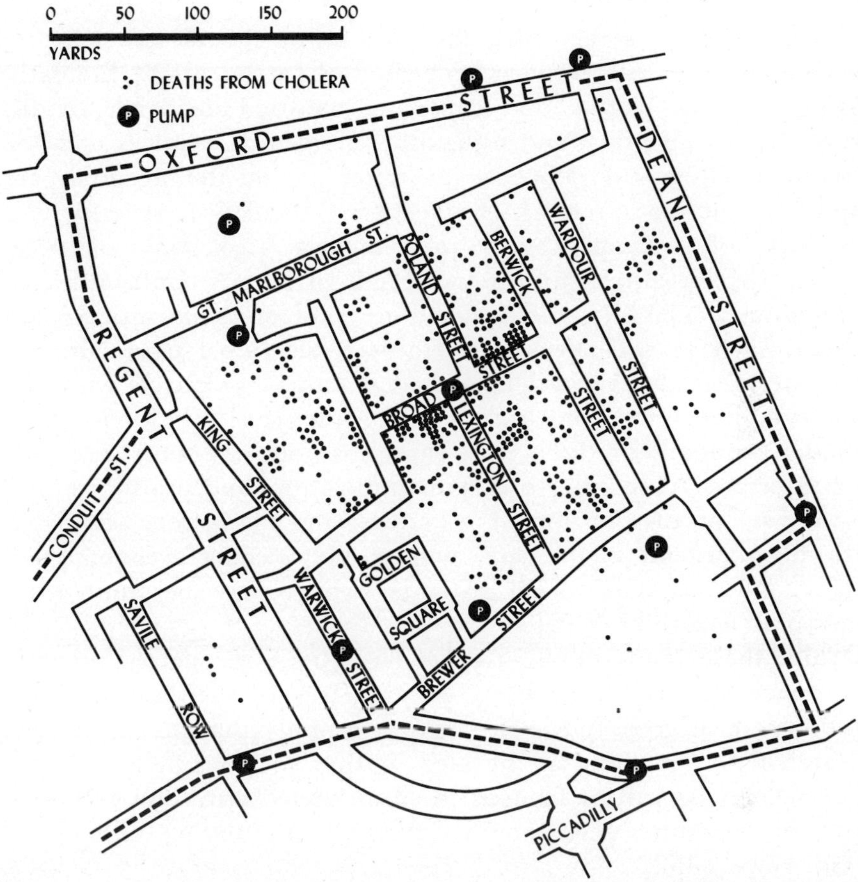

Figure 1.1. Dr. Snow's map of cholera deaths in the Soho district of London, 1848. Source: L. D. Stamp; *Some Aspects of Medical Geography*, Oxford University Press, 1964, p. 16.

appeared to cluster around a pump on Broad Street from which local residents received their water. Subsequent removal of the pump handle resulted in the termination of new cholera cases.[5]

More recent studies still rely heavily for analysis on a visual interpretation of mapped distributions; [6] however, the subject matter remains, with few exceptions, unchanged from Finke's statement above. Problems related to data in this classical approach are recognized in the report of the study group convened by the Council for International Organizations of Medical Sciences. They stated for example, that mortality data are at best a poor index of incidence and in some cases the fatality of the disease may be affected by the availability or efficiency of treatment.[8] Similarly Davies discusses factors that confound reported incidence of diseases. "The availability and utilization of medical services and the extent of supervised deliveries at home or in the hospital, are important factors affecting the recorded incidence, severity and mortality of eclampsia and preeclampsia (toxemias of pregnancy)."[8] He also mentions four kinds of factors contributing to differential availability and utilization: (1) factors intrinsic to the patient, such as socio-economic status, educational level, and beliefs and attitudes toward health; (2) factors associated with the socio-economic environment, including the level of development and the economy of the neighborhood, region, or country; (3) factors associated with education, communication, and transportation, as well as the distribution of resources; and (4) factors associated with hospital and clinic care, among them equal availability of clinics and hospitals to all patients, which may be limited by geographic accessibility.[9]

While these confounding factors have been recognized, little if any concerted effort has been directed toward their investigation within medical geography. This is not to imply that no substantive research has been done in the area or that such research is necessarily recent. As will be demonstrated in later chapters an extensive body of literature pertaining to these "confounding factors" is extant since 1852.

Medical Geography – Contemporary Approach

Medical geography is composed of two subsets: the ecological approach to the spatial distribution of disease and the spatial analysis of health behavior and planning. The former is exemplified by McGlashan's recent book, *Medical Geography: Techniques and Field Studies,* while the latter is represented by this present volume. A comprehensive health planning model should attempt to solidify both these approaches; but as stated, the thrust of this book is the geography of health care, focusing on the spatial components of the health care process and the spatial distribution of morbidity and mortality as it pertains to the health planning mode.

The treatment of morbidity and mortality in the framework of a health planning model has previously received minimal attention by investigators. Traditionally, medical geography has emphasized the spatial study of diseases and their possible etiologies, but the definition has been expanded recently to include the theory of location of medical care and future planning for it.[10]

A major effort, by Pyle, has approached the task of incorporating the traditional with the contemporary in a health planning model.[11] By integrating these approaches, Pyle provides an in-depth model to analyze urban health problems in the Chicago metropolitan area. His model has two important attributes: first, it utilizes the morbidity of the population, rather than the population per se; second it incorporates the results of analysis of the hierarchy of hospital facilities for the treatment of heart disease, cancer, and stroke. With these two features, Pyle provides an interesting morbidity-oriented locational efficiency model for the treatment of the 1980 incidence of heart disease, cancer, and stroke.

Work conducted under the auspices of the American Hospital Association provides a view very similar to that demonstrated by Pyle's study. This effort by Rosenthal applies the techniques, methodology, and analytical framework of economic theory to problems in the health care field. He explicitly states that "estimation of demand rather than of need for hospital beds was necessitated by the lack of the *morbidity data* necessary to estimate need."[12] The lack of morbidity data apparently had no effect on Rosenthal's methodology, for he made no attempt to incorporate that type of information into his allocation model. Further, no consideration was given to the spatial component of health care. We believe that the spatial component may be translated into the geography of health care and that this, in turn, is an essential component of the economics of health care.

The implication of the above statement is basic. Today, health care delivery must be viewed within the framework of systems analysis. This means, of course, that any one study should focus on selected appropriate aspects of the delivery of health care yet not attempt isolation of factors independent of other disciplines. In part, such isolation contributes to the reduced susceptibility to amelioration of the United States health care crisis. Geography, though certainly no panacea, is capable of contributing to the understanding and synthesis of major segments of the health care system. The spatial element, synonymous with the geography of health care, is an important aspect of the economic, the sociological, the epidemiological, the behavioral (psychological), and other factors that constitute the system of health care.

In order to provide an overview, Chapter II presents a discussion of health care delivery system components and a description of selected international health care organizations. Chapters III and IV pertain to the distribution of medical resources and factors in the decision location process of primary physicians. Chapters V, VI, VII, and VIII present the effects of the spatial-functional aspects of the health care system and the distribution of resources on the individuals and the institutions comprising the health care process. Specifically, Chapters V and VI deal with recipient behavior, Chapter VII with provider behavior, and Chapter VIII with selected institutional policies and problems.

REFERENCES CITED

[1] Gilbert Barnhart, "Social Design and Operations Research," *Public Health Reports,* vol. 85, no. 3, March 1970, p. 247.

[2] A. M. Davies, *The Geographical Epidemiology of the Toxemias of Pregnancy,* Charles C. Thomas, Springfield, Illinois, 1971.
H. C. McGill, *The Geographic Pathology of Atherosclerosis,* Williams & Wilkins, Baltimore 1968.
I. C. Mann, *Culture, Race, Climate, and Eye Disease: An Introduction to the Study of Geographical Opthalmology,* Charles C. Thomas, Springfield, Illinois, 1966.

[3] G. M. Howe, *National Atlas of Disease Mortality in the United Kingdom,* Nelson & Sons, Ltd., London, 1963, p. 9.

[4] R. Doll (ed.), *Methods of Geographical Pathology: Report of the Study Group Convened by the Council for International Organizations of Medical Sciences,* Blackwell-Davis, Co., 1959, p. 11.

[5] L. D. Stamp, *Some Aspects of Medical Geography,* Oxford University Press, New York, 1964, p. 15.

[6] G. M. Howe, "London and Glasgow: A Comparative Study of Mortality Patterns," in *International Geography 1972,* ed. by W. P. Adams and F. M. Helleiner, University of Toronto Press, Montreal, 1972, pp. 1214-1217.

N. D. McGlashan, "Blindness in Luapala Province, Zambia," Chapter 11 in *Medical Geography: Techniques and Field Studies*, ed. by N. D. McGlashan, Methuen & Co. Ltd., London, 1972, pp. 153-163.
[7] Doll, op cit., p. 15.
[8] Davies, op. cit., p. 26.
[9] Ibid., pp. 26-33.
[10] G. F. Pyle, *Heart Disease, Cancer and Stroke in Chicago*, The University of Chicago, Department of Geography, Research Paper Series, no. 134, Chicago, Illinois, 1971, Review by G. E. A. Dever, *Annals of the Association of American Geographers*, vol. 62, no. 3, September 1972, p. 528.
[11] Ibid.
[12] G. D. Rosenthal, *The Demand for General Hospital Facilities*, Hospital Monograph Series, no. 14, American Hospital Association, 1964.

Chapter II

SPATIAL ORGANIZATION OF HEALTH CARE:

Selected International Examples

Health care systems throughout the world have been compared for similarities and differences from several vantage points, including: economic, social, utilization, availability and accessibility.[1] The major focus of this section is the spatial organization of the various selected international examples of health care systems. The examples to be examined here include the U.S.S.R., Sweden, England, and the United States. To better understand the selected examples it is essential to briefly elaborate on the basic features of health care systems, in particular, the types of physician-patient relationship, financing, and the method of payment.

Physician-Patient Relationships

The delivery of health care was achieved in several ways before the modern development of national systems, which organized the financing and payment for medical care.[2] Physician-patient relationships within a particular country could include all or primarily one of the following types. Some were more common than others and patterns change over time. The most frequent physician-patient relationships include:

1. *Free Practitioner.* Physician relationships with the patient are exclusive and private in both the delivery of and payment for care (most frequent in the United States).

2. *Contract Physician.* Physicians contract with an association of consumers who prepay costs via subscription fees (similar to Health Maintenance Organizations (HMO) in the United States).

3. *Physicians or Officer of a Governing Authority.* Governments retain physicians for the care of patients in public hospitals (e.g., U.S. Veteran's Administration Hospitals) or practice in remote parts of the country (e.g., United States Public Health Service).

Currently, there are basically two national systems of financing and paying for medical care. They are National Health Insurance and National Health Services. National Health Insurance levies taxes on employees and their employers. The revenues are deposited in special funds and these funds, in turn, are used to pay for medical care. This is the dominant form in most European countries and in other modern nations (e.g., Sweden, Australia, and the United States—Medicare and Medicaid).

On the other hand, National Health Services revenues come from the national treasury supported by taxpayers. but every citizen by right has access. This form of financing is still relatively rare. England, U.S.S.R. and China are the principal countries in which this method is used, but it is most likely to diffuse throughout much of the world because of the heavy governmental involvement in health delivery and the high proportion of physicians in government service in developing countries.

Methods of Payment

The various systems of health delivery are clearly related to different methods of payment; for example, National Health Services can be found using any one or a combination of the several payment methods, though it tends to use the more predictable technique of salary and to avoid fee-for-service. To avoid possible confusion, it is necessary and appropriate to elaborate on each method of payment.[3]

1. *Fee-for-Service* requires payment for each medical procedure. Under *service benefits* or *direct payment* methods, the third party—that is, the sick fund or health service—pays the doctor directly, and the patient usually pays "nothing." Under *cash*

benefits or *reimbursement* methods, the patient pays the doctor and subsequently regains all or most of the fee from the third party.

2. *Capitation* establishes a fixed annual payment for each person on a list of patients regularly assigned to a doctor. The physician provides necessary care to those on the list who come to him. From a physician's viewpoint there are both advantages and disadvantages. One advantage is that, even if an individual never visits him, the doctor automatically collects the capitation fee. On the other hand, a physician usually receives only an equal capitation fee for those patients with many medical problems and frequent visits. Patients usually pay nothing directly to the doctor.
3. *Salary* provides a fixed amount of money, scaled according to the level of service and the amount of time required of the physician. Again, patients usually pay the doctor nothing; but some arrangements allow the doctor to collect fees from a third party, in addition to the salary given for required care.
4. *Case Payments* are fixed sums given the doctor for providing a patient with all necessary care on an individual case basis. They differ from *capitation* fees, which are paid for persons on a list regardless of illness. Case payments differ from *fee-for-service* in that payments are not itemized by procedure and then totaled. The few case payment systems use the *service benefits* principle: the third party pays the doctor and the patient pays nothing.

None of the above payment schemes are linked directly to any particular system of organizing a national delivery of medical services. Usually, however, the adoption of a particular payment mechanism results from a blend of national tradition and political compromise. It is ture, therefore, that the type of system and the method of payment are in some accord with tradition and politics and contribute to many of the complexities observed in health delivery systems.

Central Place Theory: A Spatial Functional Organization

Optimally, the planning of a health care delivery system should include consideration of the spatial perspective as well as the aspatial considerations mentioned above. The former include

(1) facilities: a spatial-functional hierarchy of hospitals and neighborhood clinics, including locational analysis, and delination of service areas, and (2) manpower: physicians, nursing, and paramedical personnel (i.e., distributional problems). The problems of equitable distribution and optimum location of health services may be viewed within the concept of central place theory.

One may view organization of health care delivery systems from a spatial and functional point of view. This implies a "central place" hierarchy appropriate to planning for health facilities. The spatial pattern of health care facilities in a country or region may, theoretically, range between the upper and lower limits of a hierarchical spectrum. The upper level of the hierarchy, for example, would be a large medical center providing the entire range of possible services in the designated region. At the lower level of the hierarchy, services would be provided by a ubiquitous distribution of individual physicians or paramedical personnel in an office or home-based practice. The hierarchy that is organized, or evolves, is based partly on functional organization, which reflects the fact that increasing population concentration allows greater diversity and specialization within the health services, as well as an increasing number of facilities and services to be directly related (with important exceptions) to the size of the central place. In reality the optimal organization, be it competitive or social, will have the entire range of facilities and services. "The present functional organization of facility patterns suggest that a hierarchy of facility types, defined in terms of the range of services offered and the scale of output, is desirable."[4] The present spatial organization of facilities, however, indicates varying degrees of dispersion for facilities at different levels of the hierarchy. The spatial organization is more difficult to realize because of many irregularities in the region. Such irregularities include localized resources, variation in population densities, a hierarchical transportation network, and other peculiar cultural and physical constraints that spatially distort attempts to optimize facility patterns and service areas based on theoretical considerations of an isotropic plain. Nevertheless, when health care planning decisions are being made, it is useful to think first of the "ideal" (functional and spatial) hierarchy and location pattern for an entire regional system. Distortions, due to reality, may be incorporated when specific locations are selected and when the exact nature of the population to be served is determined.

In the central place model, a flat, uniform, and unbounded (isotropic) plain is postulated. Figure 2.1 shows the resulting spa-

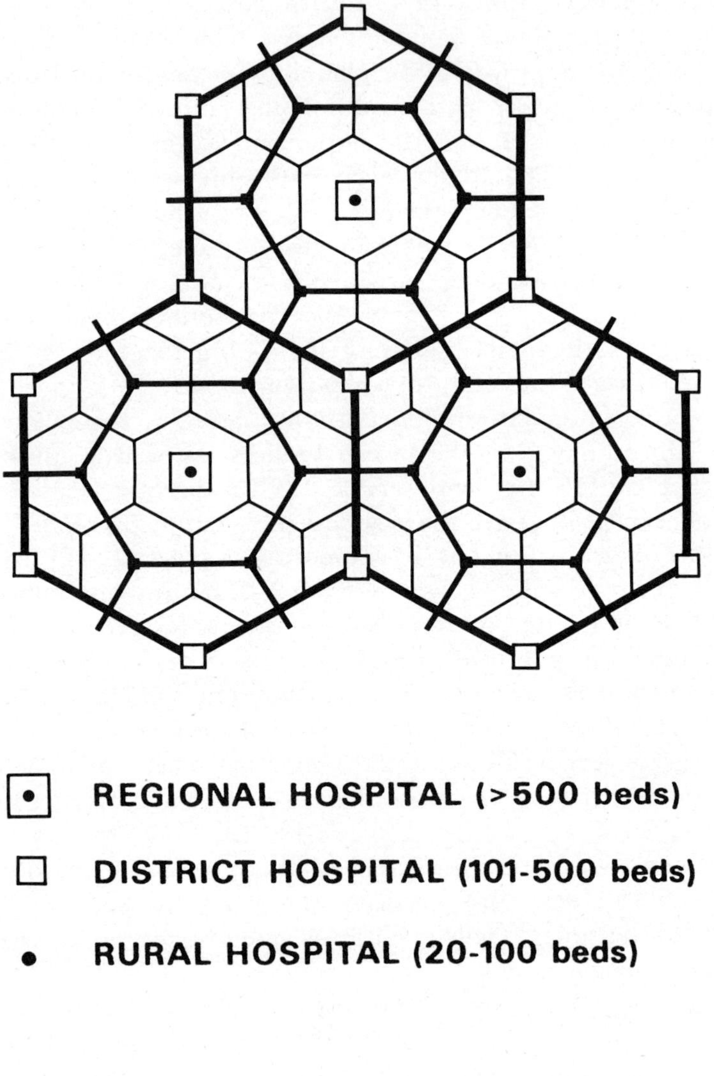

Figure 2.1. An ideal health delivery model.

tial configuration of such a model. The geometrical shape of the hexagon represents the spatial organization of the model, while the changing size of the hexagon represents the functional organization in terms of the regional development. For instance, the regional hospital, which has the largest service area and an approximate recommended bed size of greater than 500 is designed to provide complete general and specialist treatment. The district hospital, (between 101 and 500 beds), which has a smaller service area, provides fewer and less specialized services than the regional hospital but a greater number and sophistication of services than a rural hospital. The rural (local) hospital, usually 25 to 100 beds, with a much smaller service area, provides predominantly primary care in terms of general surgical and obstetrical services. It should be apparent that the optimal hierarchy (social or competitive) will vary from region to region for any country (Figure 2.2). The

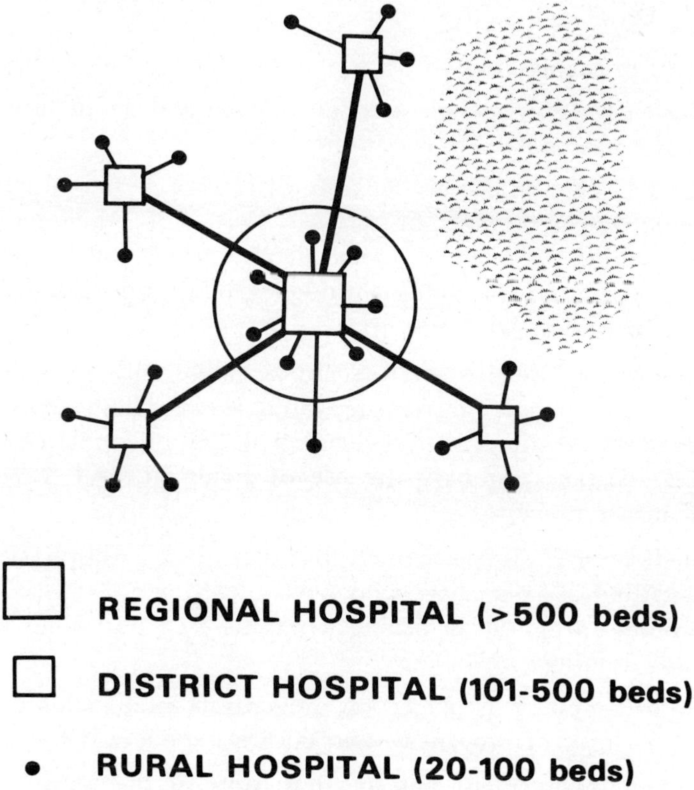

Figure 2.2 A realistic health delivery model.

variation will result from the impact of several factors including methods of payment, type of physician-patient relationships, differences in medical practice, the distribution of demand, and the type of transportation network. In order to make judgments about the applicability and desirability of central place theory as a basis for the spatial and functional organization of health services, we will examine in some detail the structural organization of selected health delivery systems.

U.S.S.R. Health Delivery System. The Soviet Union's health care delivery system has been of primary interest to health systems investigators. The interest of the U.S. researchers has stemmed from the increasing awareness of a need for a more adequate medical care system in this country. Their position has not been to argue the superiority or inferiority of the U.S.S.R. system, but simply to determine and trace the development of medical care in a socialist state.[5] The system of health care in the U.S.S.R. is premised on a number of principles:[6]

1. Health services are planned and developed as an integral part of the national socio-economic plan.
2. Medical care is free at the time of service. Nominal charges are made for a number of services (but more than half of the population is exempt from all charges). Health services are financed from the national budget (and account for 7.5 percent of the total Soviet budget).
3. Medical and health services are available and accessible to all, including people in remote, rural areas. These areas are provided for through the services of physicians or feldshers (medical assistants) and by the use of road, air, and sea transport to insure universal availability and accessibility.
4. Medical care is performed by specialists. All physicians are classified as specialists who have undergone a rather extensive training program including compulsory continuing postgraduate training.
5. Major emphasis is placed on prevention in all fields of medical care. Unity of preventive and curative services is the goal.
6. Active involvement and participation of the public is an important goal, and self-care and home medication are encour-

aged. Much of the elementary and basic health care follow-up is completed by health volunteers.

These six principles provide a framework for the delivery of health care in the Soviet Union. The basic form and structure of health care services is organized at the national administrative level. More importantly the spatial and functional organization in the Soviet Union centers upon political and population components respectively. Generally, the spatial organization corresponds exactly to the structure of central and local governments, and the functional organization is based on the population size (Figure 2.3).

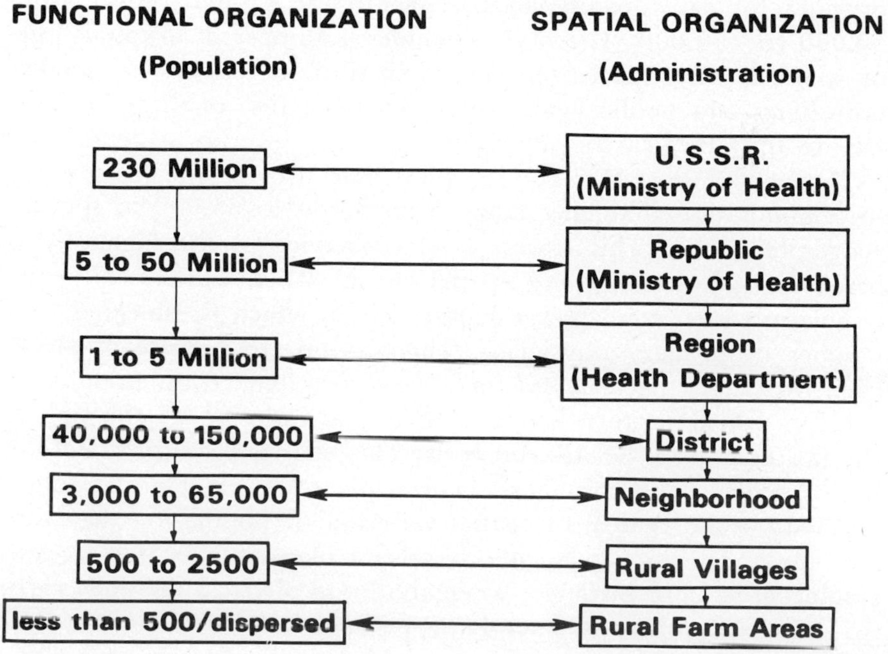

Figure 2.3. Spatial/functional organization of health care in the USSR.

The result, a most interesting feature of Soviet health care, is centralized planning. The aim is to provide centralized planning with decentralized execution.[7]

The planning of health care is coordinated centrally by the Gosplan (State Planning Committee). Under this central coordinating body, there are fifteen Soviet Republics. Each Republic has its own Ministry of Health, which is responsible for local budgeting and planning administration. The divisions within the Republics are functionally organized according to population size. The region (*Oblast*), serves populations of from one to five million. The responsibility for health services and facilities of a region is vested in an administrative appointee, the Chief Medical Officer. Responsibilities for the speciality services in the region are delegated to chiefs of the various clinical departments. Departmental chiefs are responsible for the organization and quality of work in their specialities for the entire region.

The next lower level in the hierarchy, the district (*rayon*), provides for daily maintenance of health for a population of from 40,000 to 150,000. The *rayon* includes a number of hospitals, one of which is the "specialized central institution," as well as smaller polyclinics and public health units. The direction of these facilities falls to the Chief District Physician.

The neighborhood (*uchastok*) polyclinic provides health services to a population that may range from 3,000 to 65,000 in specific geographic areas. This lowest level of service in the hierarchy is based on a functional *and* spatial organization. Functionally, the population served is approximately 4,000, which is allocated to a number of primary physicians. There is no free choice of physician. Spatially, the *uchastok* may vary according to the population density, which in turn is reflected in the variation of the size of the hospital—from 35 to 100 beds. This spatial pattern, therefore, is not typical of Christaller's central place theory, but it is more attuned to the reality of spatial variation of population densities. Specialities within the neighborhood are likewise allocated to geographic areas. For instance, a neighborhood physical therapist cares for approximately 3,000 adults; a pediatrician serves about 1,250 children under the age of fifteen; and a dentist is responsible for 2,000 or so patients. This specialty development is typical of urban medical care in the Soviet union. Thus, urban medical care is delivered at three levels: the specialized central institution; the *rayon,* or district; and the *uchastok,* or neighborhood. Further, there is a class-functional organization to the hierarchy of health services, but the spatial organization is only evident at the lowest or neighborhood level in the hierarchy.

The delivery of health care in rural areas is a rather intractable problem. Comparatively, the rural, or *rayon* (district), hospital is similar to its urban counterpart. The urban neighborhood (*uchastok*) area is replaced by a rural district concept, which serves an area of approximately 60 miles in radius and includes a similar number of people. In the more remote rural areas *feldshers* (persons trained to diagnose and treat ailments, yet not qualified doctors) are provided—one for every village or farm area. In addition, a traveling team of physicians visits the rural district hosptial (thirty beds) once a week. The *feldshers* in rural areas are responsible for primary health care of a small population—usually below 1000 persons.

Access to health services in urban and rural areas of the U.S.S.R. is provided through a range of specialists, district physicians, and *feldshers* working out of hospitals, public health units, and polyclinics. Predictably, and in accordance with the theoretical, functional, hierarchical development of central places, the larger the city the greater the degree of specialization and diversification. Thus, an implied assumption about the Soviet health delivery systems is that health care is available and accessible to all but that the quality of care varies according to the functional organization of the system; that is, increasing quality of care is associated with increasing city size.

In summary, as in all systems, there are both desirable and undesirable attributes of the Soviet health delivery system. A Health Education and Welfare report lists several of these features, which are presented below.[8] Excellent features of the U.S.S.R. system include (1) availability of health care to all; (2) emphasis on planning and frequent re-evaluation; (3) a high ratio of hospital beds, physicians, and paramedical personnel per 1000 population, the high rate of utilization; and (4) assignment of responsibility for providing health services to the polyclinic-based neighborhood (*uchastok*) physician. Selected features that might detract from the system for some include (1) the absence of free choice of physician; (2) the fragmentation of specialities into separate institutions; and (3) the assignment of physicians to "routine" duties. The U.S.S.R., as all countries, faces the problem of providing adequate rural health service. This problem is complicated by the changing manpower requirements and needs of the rural population because of their increasing desire for specialist services.

Certainly, however, centralized planning and decentralized delivery is apparent in the Soviet health system. In fact, the U.S.S.R.

has emerged as a major world leader in providing its population with equitable distribution and accessibility of health services. Essentially, the overriding feature of the system is the coupling of the political organization with the national health service. There is, however, a definite functional and spatial organization of health services, though not consistent, at all levels of the hierarchy.

Sweden – Health Delivery System. In contrast to the U.S.S.R. (and other countries–including the U.S.A.), Sweden has a rather homogenous population with respect to religion and cultural development, which provides special features and possibilities for the planning of health delivery. In addition, social policies have resulted in a health care system that is funded through a government-controlled compulsory health insurance and is supported by graduated individual taxes, fees paid by employers, and state contributions from several other revenue sources. Further, the method of payment for the provision of health service by the physician is via salary. However, as many as ten percent of the physicians remain in private practice. With these features of homogeneity, national health insurance, and salary as the method of payment, Sweden has developed an impressive plan for the delivery of health care.

Organization of medical care has a long history in Sweden, but not until 1960 was a fully organized system adopted.[9] At this time a geographer was asked to determine which cities should become regional centers for the delivery of health care. Subsequently, an in-depth study by Godlund determined, through various geographical techniques and considerations, several alternate sites for regional hospital centers.[10] The selection of each regional center was based on demographic, economic, and transportation (aggregate travel times to various centers) factors. The result of the study was the establishment of seven regional centers for the delivery of health in Sweden (Figure 2.4).

Each region encompasses three to four counties, with the populations of the regions varying from approximately 700,000 to 1,500,000. As part of this regionalization process, three questions were posed. First, what should the organizational framework be for the delivery of personal health services in a region (in order to determine the necessary regional revenues)? Second, what is the minimum (threshold) population of a region necessary to support a required specialty level of facilities? And third, a corollary of the

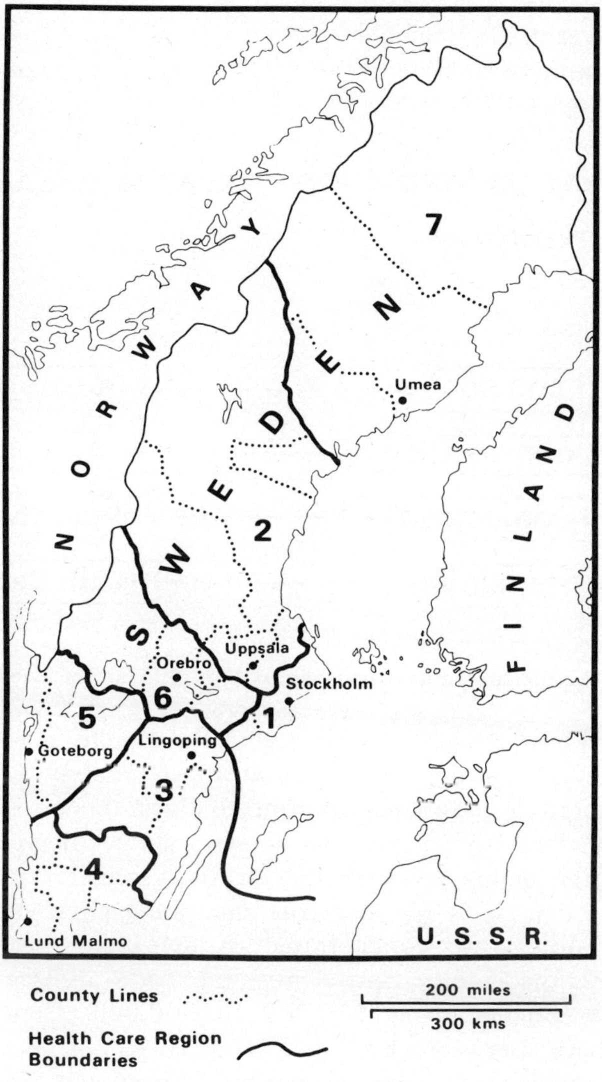

Figure 2.4. Health care regions of Sweden.

second, what is the optimum geographic size of a region to insure the maximum accessibility to the health resources for the largest number of people?[11] As a result of this planned and conditional effort to organize a regional system, spatially and functionally, a four-level hierarchical model of health care emerged (Figure 2.5).

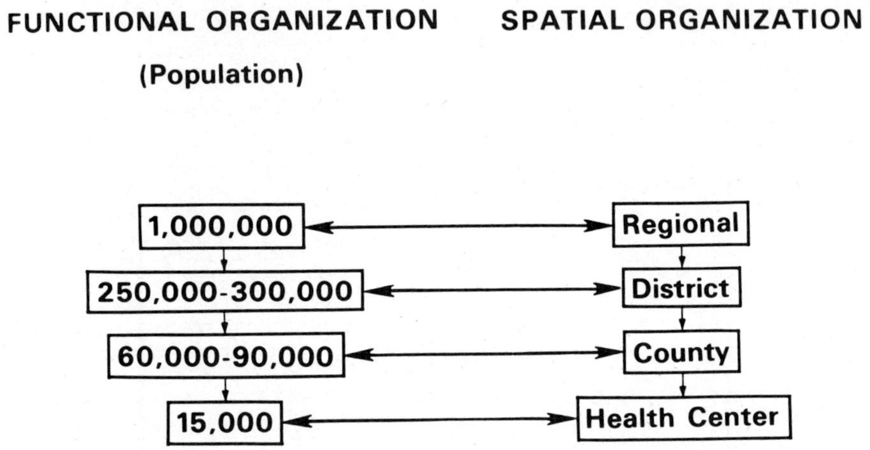

Figure 2.5. Spatial/functional organization of health care in Sweden.

At the highest level of the hierarchy, the region, a single regional hospital serves a population of from approximately 1 to 1.5 million. As noted in reference to central place theory, a functional organization based on population allows a greater degree of specialization at the higher levels in the health system hierarchy. In the case of Sweden, it is likewise true that the highest order services (super-specialities) are concentrated at the highest level. At the second level, the county central hospital serves an area containing populations ranging from 250,000 to 300,000. Generally these hospitals have between 800 and 1000 beds, all but the most esoteric specialities, a large outpatient department, rehabilitation facilities, family planning units, and welfare services.[12] The local district hospital, serving at least 60,000 and preferably 90,000 people, is the focus of the next (third) level of the hierarchy. For many years these hospitals have been an administrative problem: many are too small, serve too sparse a population, or are badly located. Swedish authorities recognize the need for converting many of these district hospitals into nursing homes, health centers, or a combination of both. As might be expected, local resistance is frequent and at times intense, but the policy remains that of eliminating all district hospitals with fewer than 300 beds. It is believed that a minimum of 300 beds is required as a threshold to support desired specialization at this level, specialization not capable of support by district hospitals with fewer beds. The lowest level of the hierarchy for medical care—the local commune (township)—is served by the health center. This health center provides ambulatory, preventive, and curative care for a population of from 10,000 to 20,000. Attached to the health center is a peripheral unit for long-term illness. However, these health centers are in the initial phase of development, and the aim is to integrate and combine their authorities with those of the nearest district hospital.

There is a functional organization of the health care system in Sweden, and its spatial organization is clearly related to the population distribution. Therefore, geographical units may very in shape and size (usually following county boundaries) to accommodate the populations to be served at different levels of the hierarchy. There is a need in Sweden, as in all other countries, to improve health delivery for the rural population. Nevertheless, Sweden has one of the most promising plans for the delivery of health care at the national level.

Stockholm: A Case Study. Stockholm has developed a unique plan for health delivery in an urban area and is most often referred to as the "classic city," which planners have suggested we use as an example of *the* "planned city." The planned system for the delivery of health care being presently implemented in the Greater-Stockholm area is scheduled for completion in 1985 (Figure 2.6). The Greater-Stockholm area will be divided into six sectors determined by the major transportation arterials that radiate out from the central city. Each sector will serve a population of 300,000 to 350,000 inhabitants. In each sector there will be one *central general hospital* located in population centers close to the main transportation line. The central general hospital is prepared to provide comprehensive services in all of the specialities of medicine.[13]

In addition, for each sector there will be two *general* hospitals providing out- and inpatient care in the basic medical practices of general medicine, surgery, obstetrics-gynecology, etc. The location

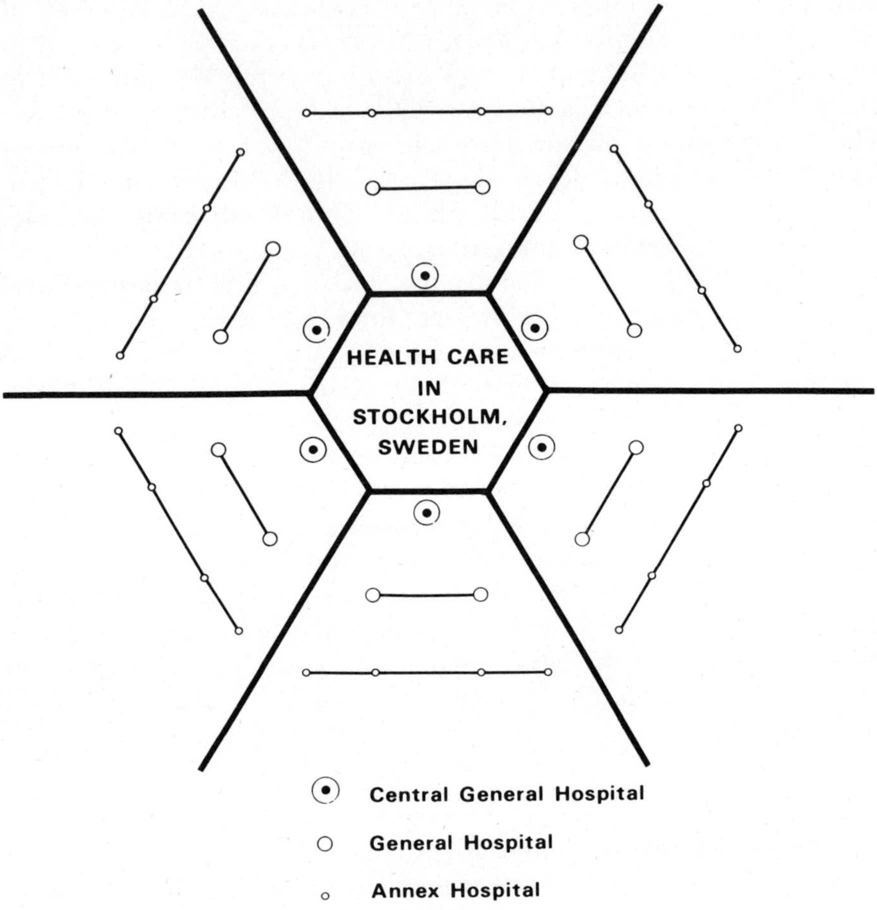

Figure 2.6. Intra-urban health delivery model.
Source: Modified after C. U. Letourneau, "Hospital Planning in Stockholm, *Hospital Management*, vol. 106, no. 4, 1968.

of these hospitals will be further away from the central city and in areas of population concentration. Beyond these two general hospitals, there will be four *annex hospitals* designed primarily for long-term and convalescent care. Each of these hospitals will have a capacity of approximately 300 beds. This intra-urban plan of health delivery is spatially organized according to the ideal health delivery model that was outlined earlier. Certainly, when this plan is realized, Stockholm will have a most progressive and sophiscated system of health care delivery.

The health care system in Sweden, however, is not without problems. In order to support their health care system and other social services, the Swedes are among the most highly taxed people in the world.[14] Lack of ambulatory care has accounted for some increased costs, and it is hoped that by encouraging provision of such care it will be possible to reduce or contain costs. The shortage and maldistribution of existing physicians present additional problems, hopefully to be overcome by building more medical schools and establishing priority areas in the distribution of doctors.[15] With this limited number of problems associated with the delivery of health care, Sweden is providing a quality of care that is not realized in most other countries of the world. It ranks first in the world in low mortality rates for infants and first in longevity for males. It appears that their guiding principle—that "quality care should be provided at the lowest acceptable organizational level of the medical care system"—has provided a level of quality that is difficult to fault.

England – Health Delivery System. England has had problems in the delivery of health care and is still struggling to systematize the organization and delivery of health services. To combat the health delivery problems in England, a "tripartite" structure was formed in 1948. This structure is probably one of the most widely criticized features of the National Health Service. Basically, the tripartite is composed of the following separate administrations: (1) primary medical care (general practice); (2) hospital medicine; and (3) local, or public health, services. With these divisions in the health service, there is little unification in delivery of health care at the regional district, or local levels.[16]

Even under the present system of administration, health care has some elements of a spatial and functional organization. At the upper level in the hierarchy there is a regional hospital that serves a "catchment area" containing between 3 and 4 million people (Figure 2.7). These regional hospitals, fifteen in all, were created by the National Health Service so that services would be provided where needed. An attempt was made to account for population distribution and the changing character of the population in order that duplication of services and of investment in services would be held to a minimum. However, the geographical boundaries and the location of the hospital within a region did not result from any basic analytical planning.[17]

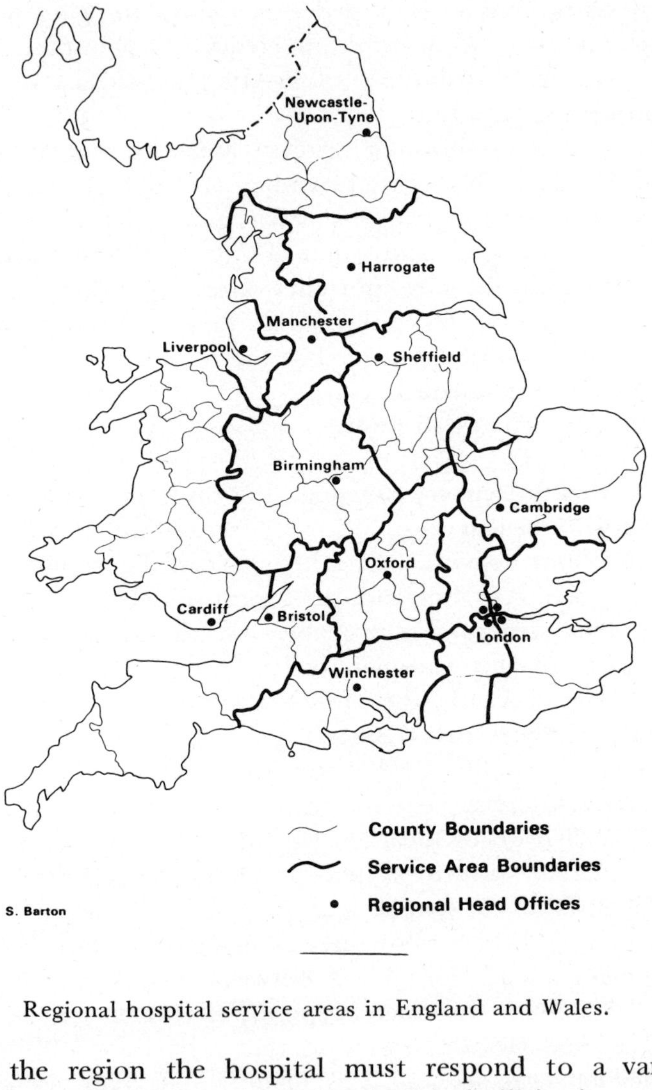

Figure 2.7. Regional hospital service areas in England and Wales.

Within the region the hospital must respond to a variety of tasks. First, an inventory of existing health facilities is required to determine future needs and projections for planning new hospital facilities. Second, an effective spatial distribution of medical manpower and allied health professions must be provided.[18] Third, at this level of the hierarchy, specialization of facilities and procedures exists.

Below the regional hospital, there is a relatively new concept in England—the district hospital.[19] In 1962, a revised health plan introduced the district hospital, which was to serve a population of approximately 100,000 to 150,000. The major purpose of this new approach was to integrate the many existing single-specialty institutions. By the late 1960s, however, the service area of the district hospital was expanded to include a population of from 200,000 to 300,000. The expansion included a greater emphasis on psychiatric and geriatric treatment, integrated planning of hospital and community health services, and a closing of the gap between hospital and general practitioner (G.P.) services by providing G.P. beds at the hospital. Before this change the general practitioner would refer a special case to a consultant, who then would be responsible for the patient; the G.P. had no access to the utilization of hospital beds. The development of the district hospital has provided some alleviation of this problem.

At all levels below the region and district, it is difficult to determine the spatial and functional organization. The difficulty arises out of the "tripartite" influence. Figure 2.8 shows the

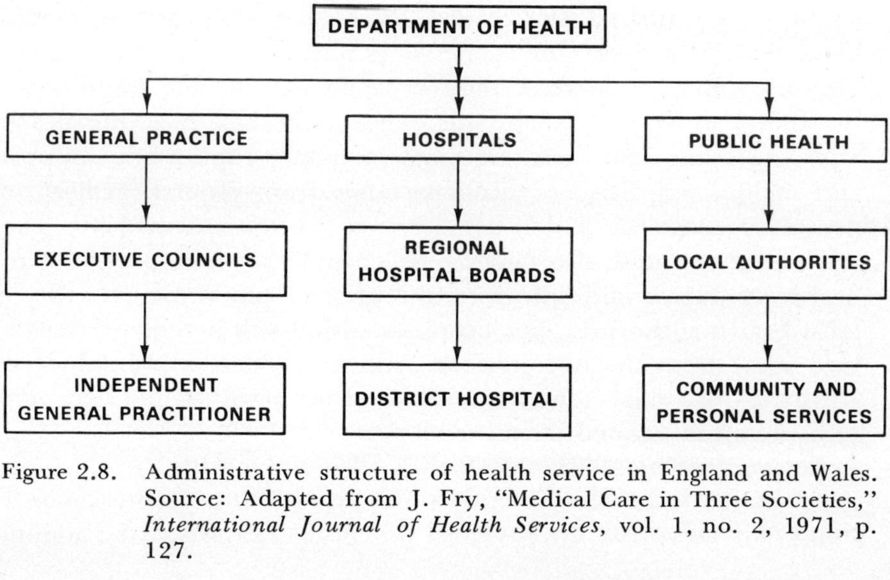

Figure 2.8. Administrative structure of health service in England and Wales. Source: Adapted from J. Fry, "Medical Care in Three Societies," *International Journal of Health Services*, vol. 1, no. 2, 1971, p. 127.

tripartite structure of health service in England, while Figure 2.9 gives a spatial interpretation of this structure. At the G.P. level, the

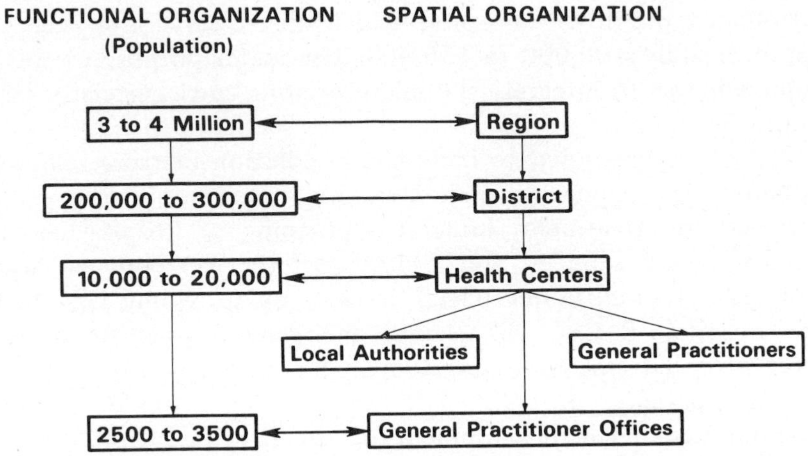

Figure 2.9. Spatial/functional organization of health care in England and Wales.

service area encompasses approximately 2500 to 3000 people. This could be considered the lowest level of health care in a quasi-hierarchy. However, the general practitioners may organize a "health center" to increase the service area to include approximately 10,000 to 15,000 inhabitants. The public health authorities are also developing health centers that are county supported, equipped, and maintained. Services available range from general medical and dental to specialist and other services for outpatients.[20] Their service area would also encompass several thousand people. Thus, health centers could integrate the general practitioners with the local health authorities, but hospitals would still be compartmentalized apart from the two services. This, in essence, could reduce the tripartite to a dual administration, and the result would be a more refined and integrated planning model.

England is "muddling through"; planning health care has been problematic since the inception of the 1948 tripartite organization.[21] There is a critical need for reorganization at the administrative level and also a need to redefine the geographical boundaries that provide the various levels of health care. The present plan is predisposed to fragmentation rather than coordination, where the services should be complementary. Two basic alternatives have been contemplated for reorganization: (1) integrate the existing structure; and (2) adopt a totally new, unified structure. To locate and allocate health services efficiently, it would be necessary for England to adopt a new plan that would encourage unification. There has, however, been resistance to this movement, and much criticism greeted such a proposal. Fortunately, it appears that England is moving toward some effective balance between centralized administration and decentralized execution in relation to the delivery of health services.

U.S.A. – A Health Delivery System? Health delivery within the United States has been labelled a "non-system system." The premise of this charge rests on the fact that health delivery has evolved and developed in a laissez faire arena and is primarily the result of local citizen desires and abilities. One could spend much time citing evidence that the American non-system of medical services is unplanned. However, it is not a non-system but a collection of several systems, subsystems, and partial systems.[22] Each system appears to be a result of conscious decision making that was limited by the concerns and perceptions of those responsible for the decisions. This lack of perception and concern, coupled with the "profit motive" as well as other considerations, forms the basis for the existing maldistribution of health services in areas such as the urban ghetto, provery-stricken rural America and—perhaps our worst disgrace—the Indian reservations.

There have been three major acts pertaining to the issue of health planning in the United States: (1) the Comprehensive Health Planning Act; (2) the Regional Medical Programs Act; and (3) the Hill-Burton Hospital and Health Facilities Survey and Construction Act. Each has been of limited value in providing a rational and equitable distribution of health resources.[23] However, a considerable range of success has been the experience in different regions of the United States. The level of success ultimately rests with concerns and perceptions of the decision makers mentioned above. Yet regardless of location, it is frequently the same social and economic groups who exert decisive control, and consequently they have determined the present aspatial organization of health services. In fact, it is ironic that the more recent discussions of national health insurance schemes have totally ignored the significance of the spatial, functional, and administrative-organizational problems that are implicit in the development of new programs. Consistently, the focus of these discussions has been on the cost of variable financing methods and the range of coverage in terms of health services. The vital concern about the multiple facets of health services delivery is eliminated.[24]

As previously suggested the American health delivery "model" is pluralistic. This model has been criticized for lack of control and coordination and has been described "as being the result of a haphazard growth of uncoordinated institutions." [25] [26] "The traditional medical care delivery system is primarily oriented toward treatment during the acute phase of illness and does not generally offer the public a complete, coordinated spectrum of health care, including the maintenance of good health."[27] This system is characterized by a maldistribution of medical services and facilities, particularly unavailable to the lower socio-economic strata of the population. Further, the system suffers from unnecessary duplication of services and facilities and unwarranted costs relative to the location and use of these facilities and services.

Alternative medical care delivery shcemes used or advocated include the following: (1) Prepaid Group Practice, (2) Medical Care Foundations, (3) Health Maintenance Organizations (HMO's), and (4) Health Care Corporations (HCC's).

Prepaid Group Practice. Prepaid group practice plans attempt to organize, finance, and deliver continuous health coverage on the basis of prepayment for a defined population. Kaiser-Permanente is currently the largest prepaid group practice in the United States. It operates with decentralized management, and each sub-region is, for the most part, autonomous. Coverage presently extends to approximately 2.3 million people in six geographic service areas: (1) Northern California; (2) Southern California; (3) Portland, Oregon; (4) Hawaii; (5) Cleveland, Ohio; and (6) Denver, Colorado. The second largest prepaid group practice plan in the United States, with a membership of about 750,000, is the Health Insurance Plan of Greater New York (HIP). Both of these plans have common principles: (1) prepayment; (2) group practice; (3) capitation rather than fee-for-service; and (4) a comprehensive spectrum of coverage. Additional aspects of the Kaiser-Permanente are (1) a unified medical center (hospital and satellite clinics) and (2) voluntary enrollment. Results of numerous studies indicate that prepaid group practice plans have lower hospital-use-rates than traditional insurance plans such as Blue Cross-Blue Shield. [28]

However, the growth of these plans has been inhibited in part by American Medical Association (AMA) opposition. The AMA position recently has been one of opposition not to the concept of prepaid group practice but to the promotion of one form of medical practice to the exclusion of others.

Medical Care Foundations. Foundations for medical care are organizations of physicians sponsored by state or local medical societies. Presently, there are some forty-six foundations distributed throughout nineteen states and thirty-two medical societies in an additional twenty-two states that are in the process of forming foundations.[29] These programs are primarily non-spatial in organization and their rapid growth may be based in part on a fear that the solo fee-for-service practice is threatened by the advent of a National Health Insurance program. Of further concern is a lack of quality and consumer control. Probably the best known, as well as the first, foundation is the San Joaquin County Foundation for Medical Care. Operating since 1954, this plan has proven to be compatible with the pluralistic systems that include the notion of prepaid group practices, Blue Cross-Blue Shield, and other (indemnity) programs, which for the most part are insufficient for specific segments of the population.

Health Maintenance Organization. Of most recent interest in the delivery of health care is the Health Maintenance Organization (HMO). Basically, an HMO has four components: (1) an organized health care delivery system that encompasses the manpower and facilities for the population to be served; (2) an "enrolled" membership that contracts for provision of services; (3) a financial plan that establishes a range of services on a prepaid basis; and (4) a managing organization that assumes accountability for all legal, fiscal, public, and professional aspects.[30] An HMO may be structured as either prepaid group practice plan or medical care foundation. Hospitalization rates are lower for both organizations than rates associated with the traditional systems of health care.[31] The paucity of comparative studies among HMO's and other health care delivery systems leaves a major void. The HMO concept is meritorious, but there is a noticeable lack of a centralized spatial organization.

Health Care Corporations. The American Hospital Association believes that a new mode of health care delivery is required. This system, Health Care Corporations (HCC), responds to the recurring problems of cost, availability, and accessibility of medical services. Its functional organization would satisfy population needs, and defined geographic areas in the United States would have at least one HCC. This system would be centrally organized with decentralized execution based on a functional relationship between population and geographic area. Such a plan, with potential to provide medical care for many indigent groups, is likely to be opposed by the AMA. Specifically, the AMA is "opposed to a rigid, centrally organized health care system" and favors "a system of private medical and health services, a pluralistic health delivery system free from centralized controls and regulations, and a voluntary approach to health care planning at the community level."[32]

Quite possibly the achievement of regional systems may evolve from the HCC's that the AHA is proposing. An example of a possible spatial/functional organization of health care delivery is that illustrated for Georgia in Figure 2.10. Regional health care systems may be systematically organized according to a spatial and functional (population) hierarchy. Regional systems did not develop earlier because of the resistance by hospitals and physicians, a resistance that stemmed from the belief that they should be free to develop *and* manage their own affairs and that the development should not be centrally directed. It was also felt that regional systems could result in services being relocated, and communities losing ready access to services have been reluctant to participate in regional systems. Thus, the 1940 theoretical base suggested by the Public Health Service (PHS) was voluntary; and the hospitals, physicians, and health planners did not direct their efforts to develop such a system. Instead, multiple systems have developed that are non-directed, uncontrolled, and changing with the changing concerns and perceptions of individuals with limited knowledge or rigid positions. The indigent population is still under-serviced, undoctored, and over-diseased.

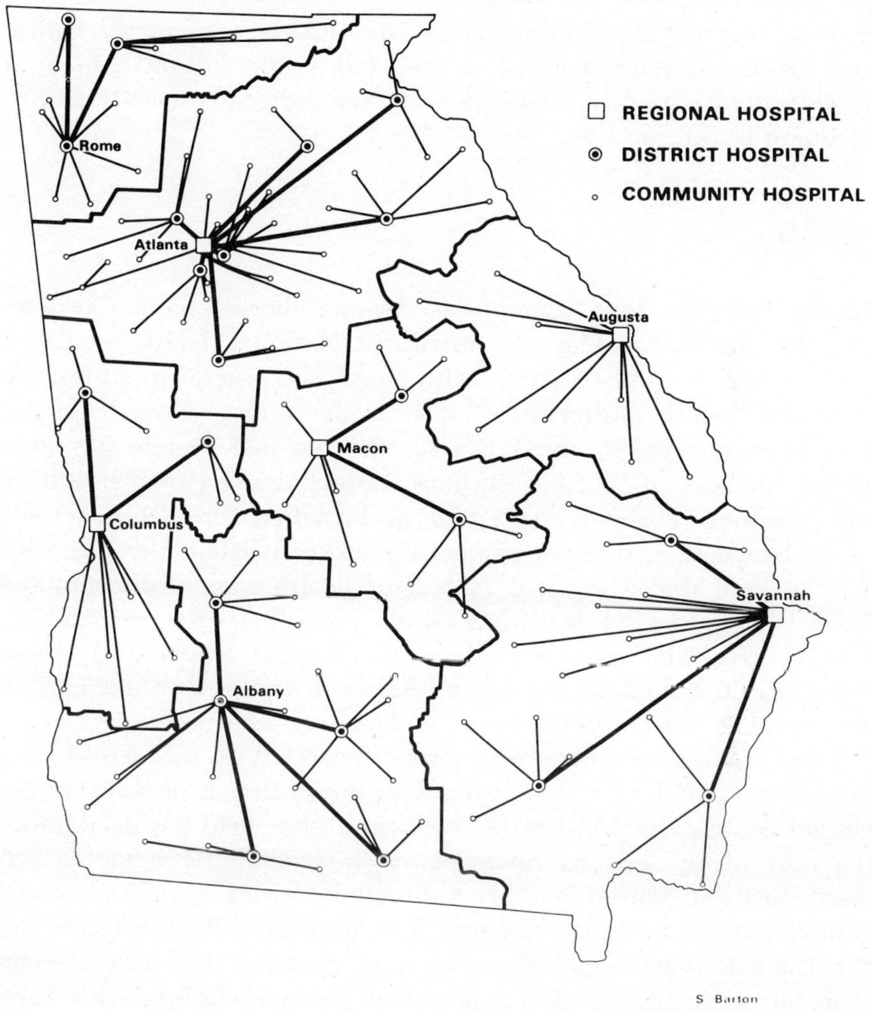

Figure 2.10. Regional health delivery model in Georgia, 1970.

The plan envisioned by PHS would establish four types of health facilities within an organized framework and determined geographical service areas. These four types included (1) base or contract hospitals, (2) district hospitals, (3) rural hospitals, and (4) community clinics. This plan is hierarchical both from a spatial, or geographical, and functional point of view. Thus, the HCC's that are being proposed are basically the same as the PHS plan to develop regional hospital systems. The HCC is particularly significant to the development of a new and viable system, which, if implemented correctly, could provide the indigent population with adequate health services.

Summary

Sweden perhaps best exemplifies regional health service systems existing in Europe today. As noted, the National Health Service of England is a regional system with hospitals, general practitioners, and local health authorities, but it is developing toward a more integrated system. In the U.S.S.R., the regional system has integrated medical or *feldsher* stations, polyclinics, regional hospitals, and teaching hospitals to assure accessibility for all geographic areas. Nowhere is it more apparent than in Sweden, the U.S.S.R., and England that a regional system of health care, if directed and funded correctly, is instrumental in providing effective, quality health care. This is reflected in the relative position of these countries compared to the United States in terms of infant mortality, maternal mortality, longevity, and death from certain diseases.

There are several points of interest that relate to problems in the organization of health care systems in the future. Especially, in the United States, the concern in the health care field has been about the cost of the various financing methods and the scope of services. Little attention has been directed toward the other crucial components of health service and their provision. Both Sweden and the U.S.S.R. have regional health care systems that have services available virtually to all segments of the population, with total national expenditure comparable to that of the U.S. England also has a regional system but it is in the midst of integrating the various parts. Evolving from the previous discussions on international health care systems are several principles that recommend themselves for development of a health care system in the United States. First and more important, some form of spatial and functional organization must be recognized as necessary for the most effective delivery of health care. Second, basic medical service should be available and accessible to all regardless of barriers such as race, income, and religion. Third, a regionally centralized administration should oversee a functionally and spatially decentralized execution of a coordinated and integrated system of medical service; these should include primary inpatient and outpatient care, dental care, and psychiatric services. Fourth, not only curative but preventive medicine as well should be required; and therefore, there is a need to understand the social and physical environments and their interrelationships. Finally, a concerted effort must be initiated to determine the health needs of the population and to eliminate the current emphasis on planning only with reference to a demonstrated demand. Some of these principles are moot points, some are generalizations, but none are principles that cannot be applied and interpreted in the United States. The future success of planning for health care organizations in the United States is dependent on the development of a basic system that is concerned with functional and spatial organization. The key to this regionalization plan is centralized administration with decentralized execution.

REFERENCES CITED

[1] J. Fry, "Medical Care in Three Societies," *International Journal of Health Services*, vol. 1, no. 2, 1971, pp. 121-133.
K. L. White, et al. "International Comparisons of Medical-Care Utilization," *The New England Journal of Medicine*, vol. 277, no. 10, September 7, 1967, pp. 516-522.

[2] W. A. Glaser, *Paying the Doctor*, The Johns Hopkins Press, Baltimore, 1970.

[3] Ibid., p. 25

[4] G. P. Schultz, *Health Care Facility Patterns for a Metropolitan Region*, Mimeo., Regional Science Group, Harvard University, 1968, p. 16. Also Discussion Paper Series No. 34, Philadelphia, Regional Science Research Institute, 1969.

[5] A. S. Yerby, "Medical Care in the Soviet Union," *Medical Care*, vol. VI, no. 4, 1968, pp. 280-285.
T. M. Ryan, "Primary Medical Care in the Soviet Union," *International Journal of Health Services*, vol. 2, 1972, pp. 243-253.

[6] J. Fry, Op. Cit., pp. 121-123.

[7] D. J. Henderson, "Soviet Medicine," *Canadian Journal of Public Health*, vol. 59, March 1968, pp. 105-110.

[8] *Hospital Services in the U.S.S.R.*, U.S. Department of Health, Education and Welfare, November 1966, PHS No. 930-F-10, pp. 4-5.

[9] American College of Hospital Administration, *The Swedish Health Service System,* Lectures from the A.C.H.A.'s 22nd Fellows Seminar, Stockholm, 1969, University of Chicago.

[10] S. Godlund, "Population, Regional Hospitals, Transport Facilities and Regions: Planning the Location of Regional Hospitals in Sweden," *Lund Studies in Geography, Series B Human Geography,* no. 21, 1961, p. 32.

[11] V. Navarro, "Methodology on Regional Planning of Personal Health Services: A Case Study – Sweden," *Medical Care,* vol. VIII, no. 5, 1970, pp. 386-394.

[12] A. R. Somers, "The Hospital is the Core of the System," *Modern Hospital,* vol. 115, no. 3, September 1970, pp. 87-91.

[13] C. U. Letourneau, "Hospital Planning in Stockholm," *Hospital Management,* vol. 106, no. 4, 1968, pp. 29-33.
L. Werko, "Swedish Medical Care in Transition," *The New England Journal of Medicine,* vol. 284, no. 7, February 18, 1971, pp. 360-366.

[14] J. Carlova, "National Health Insurance: Sweden, Where Doctors Learned to Like It," *Medical Economics,* vol. 47, September 28, 1970, pp. 102-105.

[15] L. Haanes-Olsen, "Changes in the Sickness Insurance Program in Sweden," *Social Security Bulletin,* vol. 33, no. 8, 1970, pp. 26-28.

[16] A. Smith, "General Practice Present and Future in the United Kingdom and Europe," *International Journal of Health Services,* vol. 2, no. 2, 1972, pp. 255-262.

[17] (American College of Hospital Administrators), *The British National Health Service,* 1969, pp. 19-34.

[18] D. R. Brown and T. E. Chester, "Hospital Planning in Practice: A Cross National Study," *Hospital Administration,* vol. 14, 1969, pp. 99-113.

[19] T. A. Ramsay, "New District Hospitals," *The Hospital,* July 1965, pp. 345-438.

[20] D. Owen, B. Spain, and N. Weaver, *A Unified Health Service,* Pergamon Press, New York, 1968, pp. 9-19.

[21] G. L. Maddox, "Muddling Through: Planning for Health Care in England," *Medical Care,* vol. IX, no. 5, September-October, 1971, pp. 439-448.

[22] Macy Josiah, Jr., Foundation. *The Future Role of University Based Metropolitan Medical Centers,* W. F. Fell Publisher, Philadelphia, 1972.

[23] V. Navarro, "The City and the Region—A Critical Relationship in the Distribution of Health Resources," *American Behavioral Scientist,* 1971, p. 882.

[24] D. Mechanic, *Public Expectations and Health Care,* John Wiley and Son, New York, 1972.

[25] Comptroller General of the United States, *Study of Health Facilities Construction Costs,* Report to the Congress of the United States, U.S. Government Printing Office, Washington, D.C. 1972, p. 888.

[26] Much of this discussion is adapted from the above pp. 809-888.

[27] Ibid, p. 810.

[28] E. W. Saward, *The Relevance of Prepaid Group Practice to the Effective Delivery of Health Services,* U.S. Department of HEW, Health Services and Mental Health Administration, Office of Group Practice Development.

E. Saward, J. Black, and M. Greenlick, "Documentation of Twenty Years of Operation and Growth of a Regional Group Practice Plan," *Medical Care,* vol. 6, 1968, pp. 231-244.

[29] *Study of Health Facilities Construction Costs,* op. cit., p. 819.

[30] E. W. Saward, and M. R. Greenlick, "Health Policty and the HMO," *Milbank Memorial Fund Quarterly,* vol. 1, No. 2, April 1962, Part 1, pp. 147-176.

[31] Saward et. al., op. cit., 1968.

[32] *Study of Health Facilities Construction Costs,* op. cit., p. 824.

CHAPTER III

SPATIAL PATTERNS OF HEALTH RESOURCES

The present crisis in the geographic distribution of medical care in the United States concerns both health facilities and manpower. Consequently, the distribution of hospitals, dentists, nurses, and paramedical personnel is an important consideration in any solution to the complex health care problem. A lengthy discussion of these resources is beyond the scope of this book. We have selected for our major focus, therefore, what is probably the most significant problem, the maldistribution of primary physicians. This is appropriate since, under the present circumstances, the physician constitutes the first formal link between the community and the health service system and is responsible for supervising the efforts of other workers as well.[1] The importance of the location of the primary physician would be reduced, of course, under a free-access mode of health delivery and elimination of the referral constraint. However, the present distribution of physicians, observed trends in the changing locations of physicians and various attempts to explain these trends are of particular contemporary concern. The problem becomes significantly more acute however, when we realize that we are dealing not only with a maldistribution of a health resource, but with a health resource in apparent short supply.

The Physician Shortage

There is some argument as to whether a shortage of physicians does exist. One side argues that, "assuming rational organization and an instrumental approach to medical care" the physician shortage has been overemphasized. Others, however, maintain that "there is little evidence to support the assumption that the system can be made to operate efficiently under prevailing political conditions or can be sufficiently responsive to consumer demand for more personalized care and that estimates of serious physician shortage appear realistic."[2]

Just how many physicians are necessary for good quality medical care? A recent study[3] suggests that for good quality primary medical care, approximately 133 physicians should exist for each 100,000 persons. It should be recognized that this is not the first estimate of the "required" number of physicians necessary for primary care. Various estimates of 118,[4] 125,[5] and 165[6] physicians per 100,000 population have been suggested.[7] For a current average total population of about 200 million, approximately 266,000 physicians are needed for primary medical care.[8] The report estimates that in 1966 there were approximately sixty-five non-federal physicians available for primary care per 100,000 persons in the civilian population. In 1970, there were fewer—about fifty-nine physicians per 100,000 persons. The methodology employed in the study by Schonfeld, et. al., might necessitate an upward adjustment in the number of physicians per 100,000 persons. This would accommodate an ever-decreasing supply of general practitioners. It appears, however, that even a major upward adjustment would not obscure the fact that physicians are in critically short supply. Apparently, the United States has half the number of physicians required to furnish medical care according to physician standards on the content of good medical care.[9]

Viewed in terms of a physician-population ratio (recognizing the problems attending such ratios), the maldistribution of physicians in the United States is evident at several different levels. For example, certain regions of the United States, have what might be termed (when compared against a national average) an "oversupply" of physicians, while other regions suffer a critical deficiency. Similarly, a rural-urban differential in the spatial distribution of physicians exists. Rural areas frequently suffer in terms of a lack of physician services and probably represent the most intractable problem for the delivery of health care. At the metropolitan scale, the poor and, often, black neighborhoods are almost devoid of primary physician offices.

Regional Distribution of Physicians

Within the United States considerable regional variation in the geographical distribution of primary physicians is evident (Table 3.1, Figures 3.1, 3.2, 3.3). Data obtained from the American

Table 3.1. Distribution of non-federal primary physicians, population, and physicians per 100,000 population by census region, and division for 1970*

	Primary Physicians	*% of Total*	*Population*	*% of Total*	*Physicians per 100,000*
Total	107,480	100.0	203,211,926	100.0	52.8
NORTHEAST	32,443	30.1	49,040,703	24.1	66.2
New England	7,312	6.8	11,841,663	5.8	61.7
Middle Atlantic	24,481	22.8	37,199,040	18.3	65.8
NORTH CENTRAL	26,900	25.0	56,571,663	27.8	47.6
East North Central	19,075	17.7	40,252,476	19.8	47.4
West North Central	7,825	7.3	16,319,187	8.0	47.9
SOUTH	27,645	25.7	62,795,367	30.9	44.0
South Atlantic	14,261	13.3	30,671,337	15.1	46.5
East South Central	5,074	4.7	12,803,470	6.3	39.6
West South Central	8,310	7.7	19,320,560	9.5	43.0
WEST	21,142	19.7	34,804,193	17.1	60.7
Mountain	4,087	3.8	8,281,562	4.1	49.4
Pacific	17,055	15.7	26,522,631	13.1	64.3

*Primary physicians are those in the fields of General Practice, Internal Medicine and Pediatrics.

Source: J. N. Haug, G. A. Roback, B. C. Martin, *Distribution of Physicians in the United States, 1970,* Center for Health Services Research and Development, A.M.A. Chicago, 1971, and *General Population Characteristics,* U.S. Summary 1970, U.S. Dept. of Commerce, Bureau of Census, Washington, D.C.

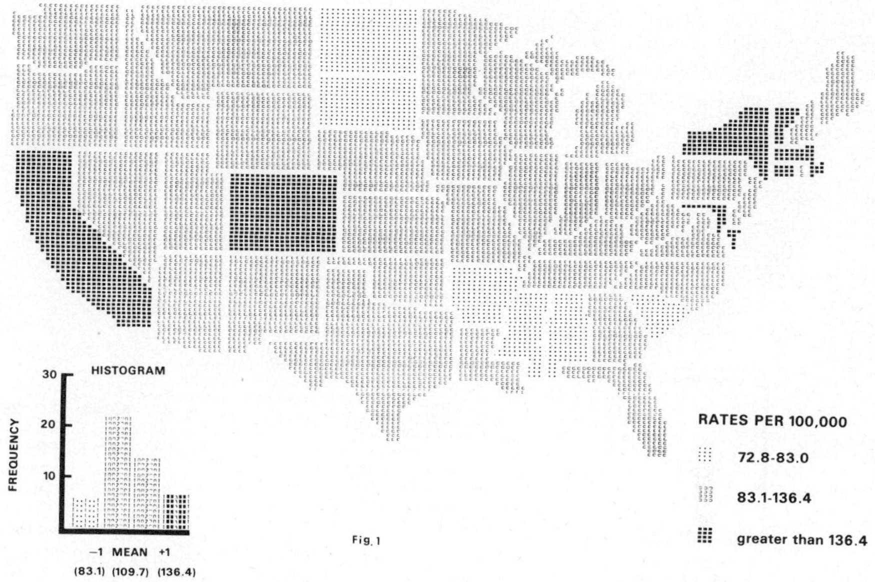

Figure 3.1. Medical resources: general practitioners, 1970.

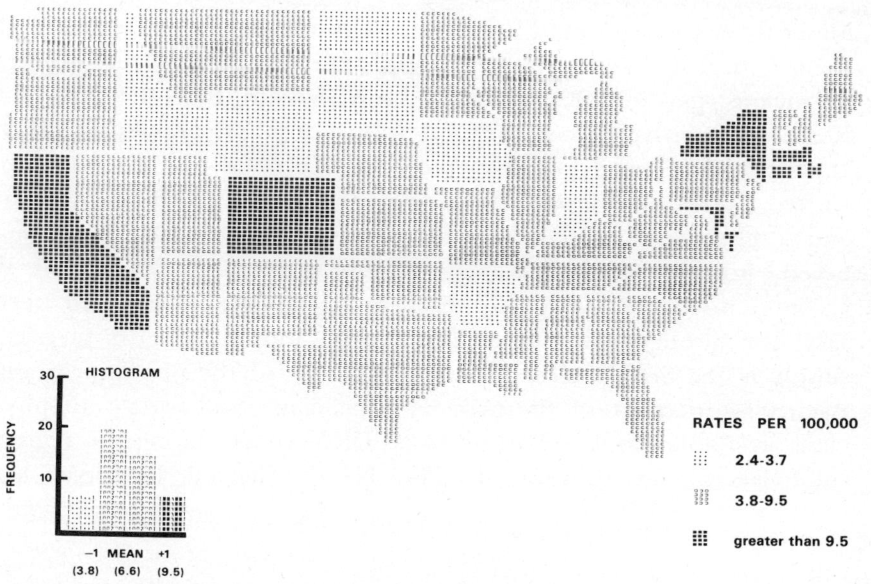

Figure 3.2. Medical resources: pediatricians, 1970.

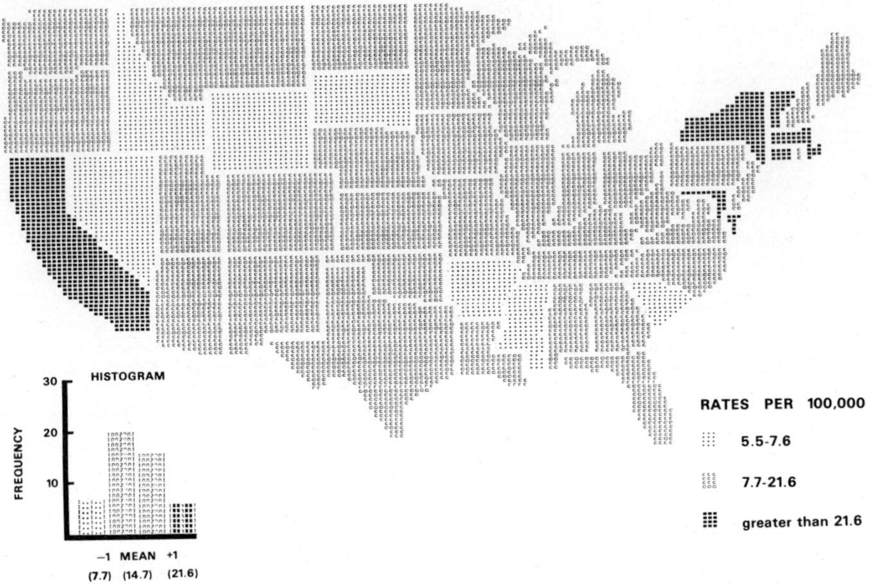

Figure 3.3. Medical resources: internists, 1970.

Medical Association[10] and the United States Bureau of the Census indicate the existence of approximately fifty-three* primary physicians per 100,000 persons. It is evident that the Northeast Region is relatively "well-off" in terms of physician supply. It has approximately twenty-four percent of the total population of the United States, thirty percent of the total active primary physicians, and a physician-population ratio of sixty-six. It must be remembered, however, that this still represents only about half of the recommended number (133) of primary physicians believed necessary for good quality care. The largest deficit area of physician supply is the South with thirty-one percent of the population, only twenty-six percent of the primary physicians, and forty-four physicians available per 100,000 persons. Differences among the regional subdivisions are substantial. The North Central Divisions have

*The study of Schonfeld, *et. al.*, indicates just under fifty-nine physicians per 100,000 persons. The discrepancy between the figures is not immediately discernable, nor is it large enough to cause concern.

almost identical physician-population ratios (47.4, 47.9), while a greater difference exists amont the Divisions of the Northeast (66.2), 61.7, 65.8) and South (46.5, 39.6, 43.0). The Mountain and Pacific Divisions of the West demonstrate a tremendous range in the number of physicians available, the former having forty-nine and latter having sixty-four physicians per 100,000 persons.

The East South Central Division, with under forty physicians per 100,000 persons has the lowest physician population ratio in the country. It is interesting to note that in 1953 the president of the State Medical Association of Mississippi was fearful (with a physician per 100,000 population ratio of approximately seventy, including all physicians) of an over-abundance of physicians to serve the people. This was due at least in part to the unelaborated fact that "Our population is peculiar in that the Negro constitutes nearly half the total population."[11] As recently as 1966, the executive secretary of the same organization stated that those who present statistics to show physician "shortages" are "very bad statisticians or out-and-out prevaricators" and "prophets of gloom, doom, and physician shortages." It [a physician shortage] never was true and patently cound not be true today."[12] Today the primary physician-population ratio for Mississippi is approximately 37.

There is also considerable variation in the locational characteristics of physicians classified as "primary." Unlike the general practitioners, the pediatricians and internists are concentrated primarily in the North East, with a minor concentration in a few of far western states. Figures 3.1, 3.2, and 3.3 show the differences in the spatial patterns of these physicians. It is apparent that high income and urbanization are centripetal forces that attract the more specialized pediatricians and internists. In addition, the geographical distribution of general practitioners exhibits a pattern of considerable interest. It may be noted, in Figure 3.1, that general practitioners are concentrated in the Midwest and in the far western states. Both groups, however, the more specialized primary physicians and the general practitioners, are avoiding most of the southeastern United States. A scale change would indicate a greater disparity in rural-urban differentials of these two groups. These patterns reflect the inequity of delivery of health care in the United States. It is most inadequate for poor black and rural populations. While the spatial distribution of the primary physician is a major concern to the delivery of health care, there are other health resources of importance, including dentists, paramedical personnel, and health facilities.

Comprehensive health care has been the goal for many of the existing and new health care programs. Without question, however, dental care is the last service to be implemented. Consideration must be given the dentists. Figure 3.4 suggests that implementing

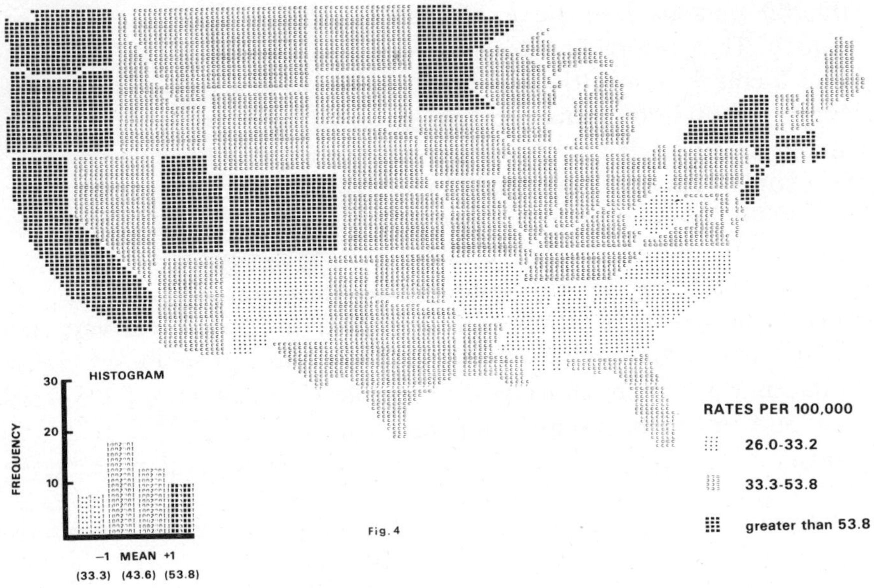

Figure 3.4. Medical resources: dentists, 1970.

such services will meet with considerable problems. For instance, the southeastern United States is grossly under-serviced, critically so in terms of developing dental care programs. From our own experience in Georgia, the rural-urban dentist differential is more severe than the physician differential.

Paramedical personnel, an increasingly important health resource commodity, is also shown to have peculiar geographical distributions depending on the specific groups. Lay mid-wives, medical technologists, and medical laboratory technicians are concentrated in the southern and southeastern sections of the United States (Figures 3.5, 3.6, 3.7). These three groups provide service in many

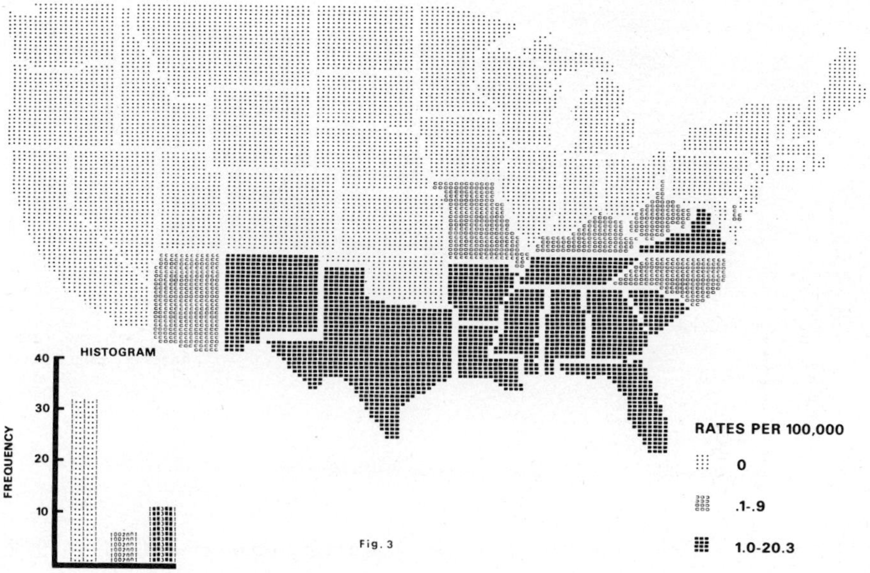

Figure 3.5. Medical resources: lay midwives, 1970.

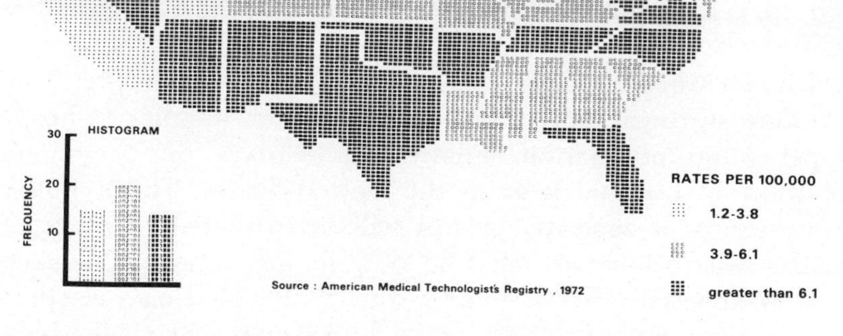

Figure 3.6. Medical resources: medical technologists (AMT), 1972.

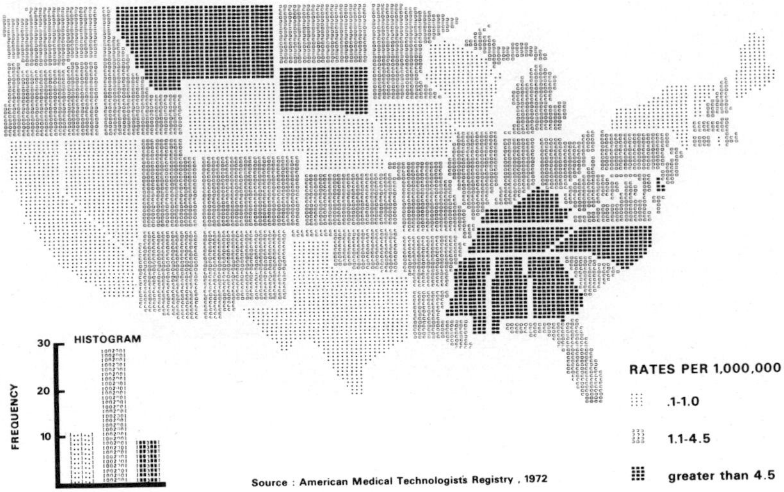

Figure 3.7. Medical resources: medical laboratory technicians (AMT), 1972.

of the rural areas. Registered nurses (Figure 3.8), likewise a key element in the delivery of health care, are concentrated in the mid-western and western states. This particular distribution is in contrast to the other three paramedical groups but similar to the geographical distribution of general practitioners. Clearly, a substitution, or trade-off, exists between lay mid-wives and registered nurses. The substitution of various paramedical personnel may create variations in the quality of health care that are functionally related to centripetal forces to be discussed in a subsequent section.

Health facilities are also unevenly distributed in the United States. One surrogate for health facilities is the number of hospital beds per 1000 population. Figure 3.9 displays the geographical distribution of hospital beds in the United States. The hypothesis that physicians or specialty groups will be attracted to a hospital, no matter where located, must be viewed with considerable skepticism. It is apparent that a comparison of the physician or specialty group maps with the hospital facilities map will challenge this hypothesis.

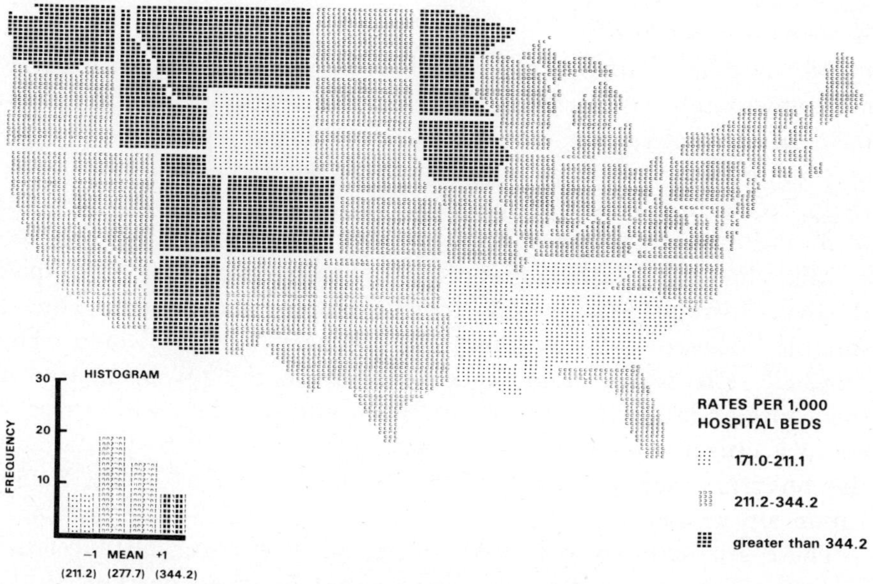

Figure 3.8. Medical resources: registered nurses, 1970.

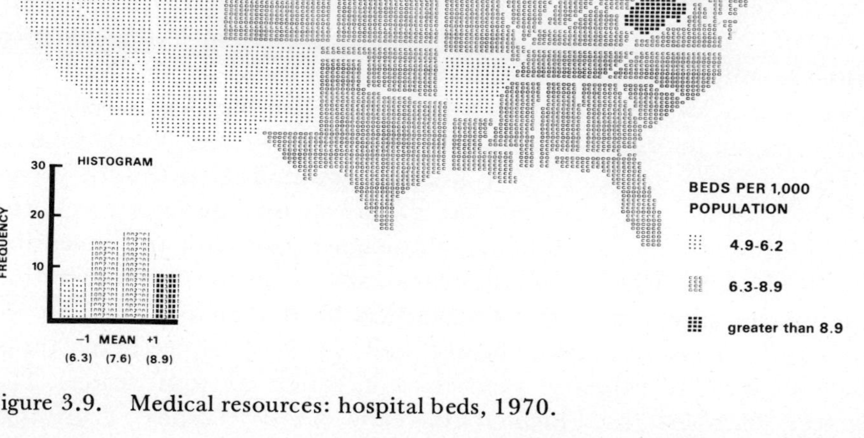

Figure 3.9. Medical resources: hospital beds, 1970.

The Distribution of Women Physicians

A man and his son are travelling down the highway in an automobile and are subsequently involved in a serious accident. They are immediately transferred to the emergency room of the nearest hospital. The physician on duty, when seeing the man and his son, says immediately, "I can't work on this case, I'm directly related to them." Question: What is the relationship of the physician to the man and his son? Generally, if you're like most, your answers include the man's father, grandfather, brother, or some other male relative. Infrequently is any female relative mentioned. Thus a suitable answer such as "mother" is very rarely offered. This "riddle" reflects the dominance of males in the physician role in the United States. If the same situation and question were presented to a citizen of the U.S.S.R. the response would be predictably the reverse, since seventy percent of the physicians in the Soviet Union are women.

There are within the United States, however, over 21,000 active women physicians comprising approximately seven percent of the total number of active physicians.[13] Perhaps more important, approximately forty-five percent (8,776) of the total number of women physicians are involved in primary medical care (Table 3.2). Women primary physicians are concentrated (Figure 3.10) in the Middle Atlantic Division of the Northeast Region (31.9%). Most of the remaining women physicians are located in the highly urbanized East-North Central Division, South Atlantic Division, and Pacific Divisions of the North Central, South, and West Regions, respectively. The comparison of Table 3.2 with Table 3.1 (Distribution of Non-Federal Primary Physicians) indicates that women primary physicians are more highly concentrated in the Northeast Region and Middle Atlantic Division than are physicians generally. They are under-represented to some extent in the North Central Region (27.8% versus 21.5%) and the South Region (30.9% versus 20.8%). However, when viewed at the census division level, the distribution of women primary physicians again with the exception of the Middle Atlantic Division generally parallels the distribution of primary physicians. The distribution by Region and Division are deceptive, however, since nearly half (47.5%) of all active non-federal women primary physicians practice in four states. The largest numbers are located in New York (1,735), California

Table 3.2. Distribution of non-federal women primary physicians by region and division for the U.S., 1970

	Women Primary Physicians	*% of total Women primary Physicians*	*Female Population*	*Women primary Physicians per 100,000 females*
Total	8,200	100.0	109,025,115	7.5
NORTHEAST	3,215	39.2	23,135,853	13.9
New England	597	7.3	5,922,912	10.1
Middle Atlantic	2,618	31.9	17,212,941	15.2
NORTH CENTRAL	1,763	21.5	26,619,635	6.6
East North Central	1,400	17.4	18,624,744	7.5
West North Central	363	4.4	7,994,981	4.5
SOUTH	1,703	20.8	25,939,667	6.6
South Atlantic	1,017	12.4	12,391,798	8.2
East South Central	255	3.1	5,232,351	4.9
West South Central	431	5.3	8,315,518	5.2
WEST	1,519	18.5	16,664,980	9.1
Mountain	208	2.5	4,009,095	5.2
Pacific	1,311	16.0	12,655,885	10.4

(1,094), Pennsylvania (552), and Illinois (506). The low representation of women in the medical profession as well as the high percentage of existing numbers of women physicians involved in primary care suggest that a partial solution to the lack of primary care man- (woman-) power could be alleviated by medical schools emphasizing recruitment among women.

Under-representation of women in physician ranks is obviously important in terms of equality of opportunity. Perhaps more important and difficult to assess is the impact of this differential in terms of the overall health behavior of women; that is, how does the prospect of being treated by a male physician contribute to the therapeutic behavior of women? Does it delay response to recognized symptoms of certain illnesses or diseases? On the other hand, is there a difference in a male and female physician's ability to understand problems of the opposite sex and consequently in their ability to treat the "whole" patient rather than just alleviate the manifest symptoms? If there is a difference, how important is it? These and related questions are being raised more frequently and suggest an appropriate area for investigation.

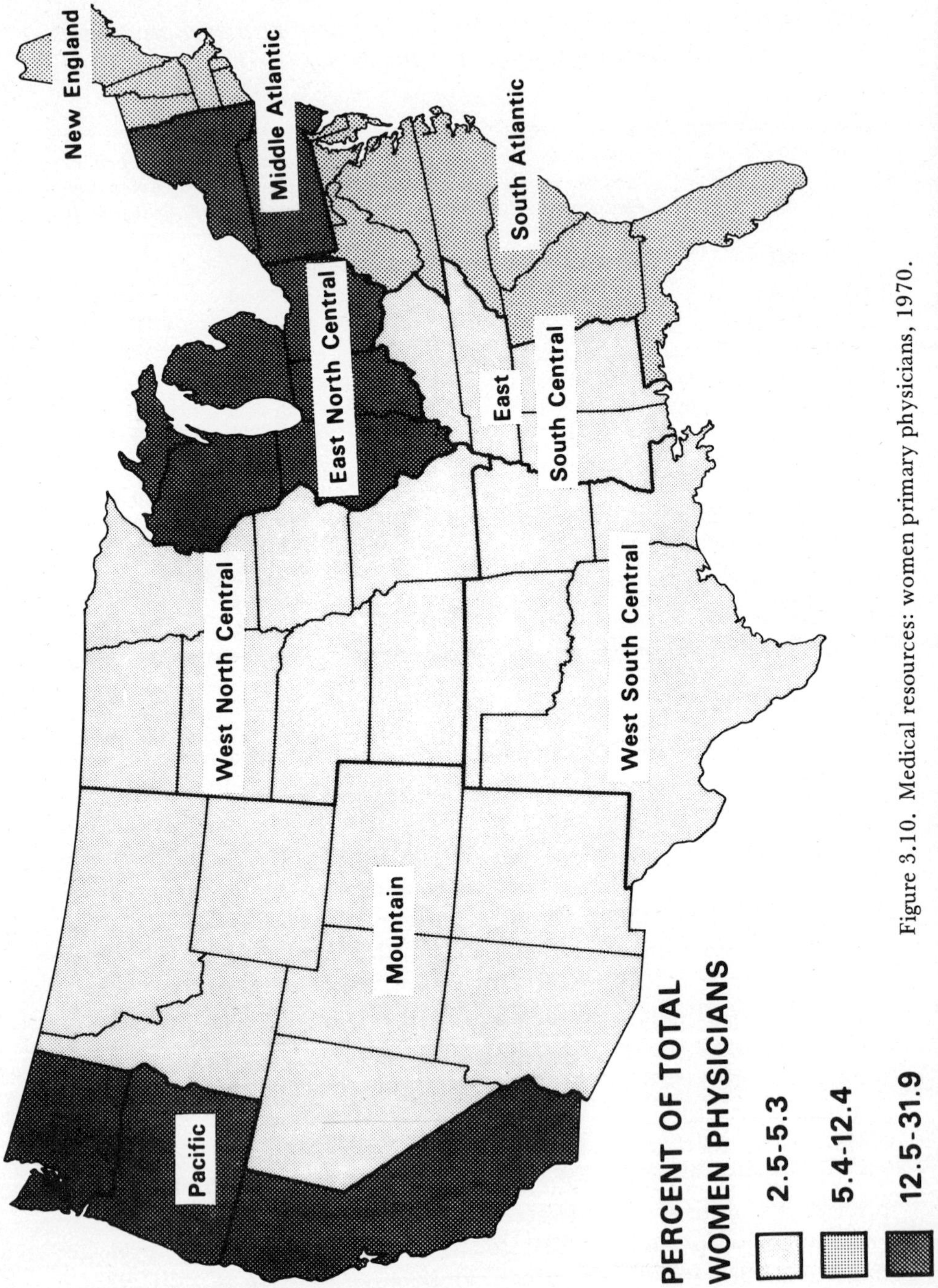

Figure 3.10. Medical resources: women primary physicians, 1970.

Distribution of Black Physicians

Functional-attitudinal studies among physicians are rare. These are studies, however, for which some illustration exists for physician attitudes. While these attitudes have never been systematically studied, there are suggestions that considerable prejudice exists among physicians toward the poor and blacks. One of the authors, in a conversation with a pediatrician was informed that "they" were notorious in missing appointments at a newly constructed clinic built especially for "them." In addition, when "they" finally showed up "they" lied in reporting reasons for missed appointments. When asked if any systematic attempt had been made to determine the reason(s) for the high percentage of missed appointments and methods by which the problem might be alleviated, the physician replied that the "board" would never consider social science intervention into the health delivery process. Evidence supporting this prejudice may be gleaned from reports of physicians' attitudes toward the poor. As discussed in Elesh and Schollaert,[14] in a random sample of U.S. physicians, conducted by mail over forty percent responding indicated that a *"dissolute* way of life is the cause of many diseases among the poor." Another study, which substantiates our conversation with the clinic pediatrician, found that generally physicians considered the poor to be dirty, smelly, *unreliable with respect to appointments and directions,* observing poor health practices, and living in unhealthful conditions.[15]

The entire problem does not rest with the provider. In each case the patient must also identify to some degree with the physician to facilitate communication. Perhaps the socio-cultural gap, such as the one between women patients and men physicians, is at least as great when we are speaking of the relationship between a physician and a poor, black patient. To facilitate treatment, it is necessary that a physician be familiar with the vocabulary and life styles of the patients. It is most important then to consider the number and distribution of black physicians, because they are also most likely to be familiar and sympathetic to the particular problem of delivering health care to those trapped in both the rural south and the inner cities.

The black population comprises approximately fourteen percent of the total U.S. population. In 1967 the number of black physicians comprised two percent (4,805) of all physicians.[16] Of these, over fifty-five percent (2,687) may be classified as providing primary medical care. A regional distribution of black physicians by specialty is not available. Generally, however, the black physicians are concentrated (Table 3.3) east of the Rocky Mountains in

Table 3.3. Distribution of black physicians (1967) and population (1970) by census region and division of the United States

	Black Physicians	*% of Total*	*Total Population*	*% of Total*	*Black Physicians per 100,000 Blacks*
Total	4,417	100.0	22,580,289	100.0	19.6
NORTHEAST	1,069	24.3	4,344,153	19.2	24.6
New England	93	2.1	388,398	1.7	24.0
Mid-Atlantic	976	22.1	3,955,755	17.5	24.7
NORTH CENTRAL	1,118	25.2	4,571,550	20.3	24.5
East North Central	921	20.9	3,872,905	17.2	23.8
West North Central	197	4.3	698,645	3.1	28.2
SOUTH	1,603	36.3	11,969,961	53.0	13.4
South Atlantic	1,084	24.5	6,388,496	28.3	16.9
East South Central	275	6.3	2,571,291	11.4	10.7
West South Central	244	5.6	3,010,174	13.3	8.1
WEST	627	14.0	1,694,625	7.5	36.9
Mountain	29	.5	180,382	.8	16.1
Pacific	598	13.5	1,514,243	13.5	39.5

Source: M. A. Haynes, "Distribution of Black Physicians in the United States 1967," *J.A.M.A.*, vol. 210, no. 1, 1968, pp. 93-95, and *General Population Characteristics*, United States Summary 1970, U.S. Department of Commerce, Bureau of Census, Washington, D.C.

the Northeast, North-Central and Southern Regions of the United States (Figure 3.11). The greatest percentage (36.3) is located in the Southern Region. The heaviest concentration appears to be in the South Atlantic, Mid-Atlantic and East-North Central Divisions (24.5%, 22.1%, and 20.9% of the total black physicians respective-

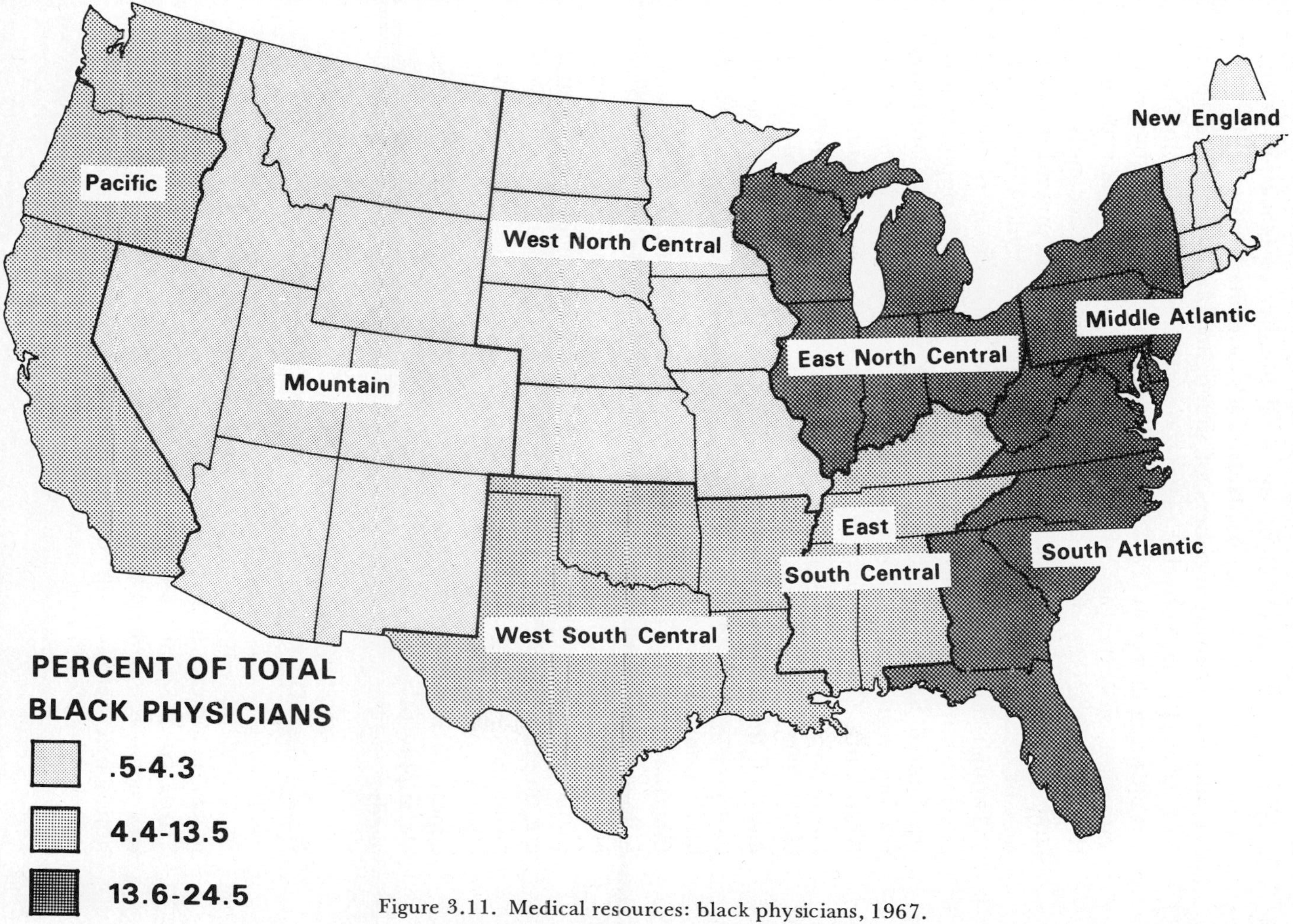

Figure 3.11. Medical resources: black physicians, 1967.

ly). In contrast the New England and Mountain Divisions contain only three percent (122) of the total number of black physicians. At the state level California, New York, and the District of Columbia have the greatest numbers of practicing black physicians (574, 562, and 417 respectively). The concentration of black physicians in California and New York is apparently the result of a substantial migration, since neither of these states trains a significant number. Howard University located in Washington, D.C., accounts for a large proportion there. An intensive survey of the present distribution of black physicians is currently being conducted.[17]

Though the South has the largest percentage (36.3) of the black physicians it contains over half (53.0) the total black population of the United States. The black physician-population ratios are lower for this region than for any other section of the nation. In the West-South Central Division, for example, the average number of black physicians available to serve 100,000 blacks is just over eight (8.1). The average ratio for the entire region is 13.4. Throughout most of the nation, with the exception of the Pacific Division, the number of black physicians does not reach thirty for each 100,000 black population. It is not surprising, as will be demonstrated later, that the rural blacks are the least healthy segment of our society, followed closely by the urban black population. It should be emphasized that, if it is important to reduce the socio-cultural-sexual gap to facilitate treatment, then the women of the nation are in the unenviable position of having the least numbers of physicians available. The highest number of women primary physicians per 100,000 women is just under fifteen (14.7). Both groups appear to be placed at severe disadvantages in terms of an equitable supply of physicians perhaps most responsive to their particular needs.

Rural-Urban Distribution of Physicians

As in the past, today many people feel that life in the country is highly beneficial to health and that those fortunate enough to live "close to the soil" are prey to less illness and consequently have less need of medical services than urban dwellers. In the early nineteenth century, in the early stages of industrialization and metropolitan evolution, this was undoubtedly true, as the residential congestion and lack of public health infrastructure contributed to disease and illness peculiar to cities. This attitude is reflected in an early (1837) statement of Dr. Benjamin N. McCready:

> Agriculture is the oldest, the healthiest, and the most natural of all employments. The husbandman, in general, enjoys pure air, and varied and moderate exercise. In this country his diet is always abundant and nutritious and his habits much more temperate than those of the manufacturing or laboring classes. His diseases commonly are acute, and are incident to an active and vigorous constitution, and he is free from the majority of nervous and dyspeptic ailments so prevalent in large cities.[18]

During this same era there was no technological inducement for physicians to favor urban settlement, nor did cities represent concentrations of wealth where a physician's income might be maximized. Add to these factors the prevalence of a rural background of most physicians, and it is evident why the distribution of physicians between town and country was probably not noticeably uneven through most of the nineteenth century.[19]

During the period from 1870 to 1910 the percentage of the total population living in urban areas rose from 25.2 percent to 45.7 percent.[20] At the same time a number of centripetal forces developed contributing to the concentration of health manpower and facilities in the cities: (1) public health services and facilities were financed through the increasing wealth of urban areas; (2) the rising per capita income of the urban dweller provided greater income potential for urban physicians relative to his rural counterpart; (3) advances in medical science increased the physicians dependence upon hospitals, their technical equipment and auxiliary personnel—capable of support only by urban centers; (4) the rising costs for a medical education restricted the majority of students to sons of wealthy urban families. These factors combined with the urban location of most medical schools did not predispose graduates to settle in country villages.[21] In addition, measures were undertaken to restrict the number and increase the quality of medical graduates, so as not to "overcrowd" certain areas.[22]

These forces, recognized as early as 1906, contributed to a rural-urban differential in physician distribution. It was estimated at this time that rural communities contained fifty-three percent of the total population of the United States and forty-one percent of the physicians.[23] By 1929, the rural communities included forty-eight percent of the population but only thirty-one percent of the physicians.[24]

In a study of upstate New York,[25] the physician population ratio in rural areas, initially lower than in urban communities, declined by twenty-three percent from 1930 to 1950. The ratio for urban communities increased by eighteen percent during the same period. It was noted in the same study that the trend toward the "disappearance of the rural physician is continuing not only in Missouri and Kansas, Louisiana and Mississippi, but also in New York."[26] Moreover, "the decrease in the number of rural physicians must be recognized as a universal long-term trend."

In the New York study, it was discovered that the urban areas were generally increasing in the total number of physicians. However, intra-urban low economic areas were actually decreasing in the number of physicians per 100,000 population. For example, during the period from 1930 to 1950, the number of physicians per 100,000 persons decreased by seven percent in the low income area of Rochester, by fourteen percent in Syracuse, and by twenty-four percent in Buffalo. A hypothesis that the decrease in physicians within these areas might be offset by an influx of osteopaths and chiropractors was not supported. On the contrary, it was found that the osteopaths located in predominately upper-income areas and areas of physician clusters.[27]

The depletion of physicians in rural areas of the Rochester region, one area included in the earlier study of upstate New York is illustrated in Table 3.4. This problem is not peculiar to the highly urbanized Northeast but is common to all parts of the nation. For example, the steady decline in the percentage of rural mid-west Iowa's farm population (Figure 3.12) has been accompanied by an apparent decision of many rural Iowa physicians to move to the larger towns and cities, as is indicated by the sharply decreasing physician-population ratios experienced by the rural areas relative to the more urbanized places (Table 3.5).

It is also apparent, as indicated by increasing average age of practicing physicians (Table 3.6), that recent graduates, have selected to enter practice in major towns and cities.[28] In 1960, the majority of physicians practicing in rural villages were over sixty years of age. On the basis of age alone, a significant natural attrition of rural physicians can be expected. The avoidance of rural areas by almost all new graduates, coupled with this natural attrition rate, projects a severe medical care crisis for rural farm populations.

Table 3.4. Ratio of physicians to 100,000 population for counties of Rochester region, N.Y., 1905-1970

	Year			
County	*1905*	*1920*	*1940*	*1960*
Allegany	116	169	171	76
Chemung	175	129	117	120
Livingston	160	111	117	64
Monroe*	112	120	131	185
Ontario	177	151	137	132
Orleans	142	125	126	53
Schuyler	214	130	92	80
Seneca	145	110	89	53
Steuben	145	125	105	93
Wayne	135	121	117	74
Yates	116	169	171	76

*Rochester Metropolitan Area
Source: R. C. Parker, R. A. Rix and T. G. Tuxill, "Social, Economic and Demographic Factors Affecting Physician Population in Upstate New York," *New York Journal of Medicine*, March 1, 1969

Table 3.5. Physician-population ratios for Iowa in counties ranked by degrees of rurality, by decade, 1910-1960

Proportion of Population that is Rural in Respective Counties	*Physicians per 100,000*					
	1910	*1920*	*1930*	*1940*	*1950*	*1960*
80% or more	148	124	99	196	71	53
60–79	168	142	112	103	85	63
40–59	154	160	141	138	124	82
Less than 40	187	165	137	125	110	105

Source: J. C. MacQueen, "A Study of Iowa Medical Physicians," *Journal of Iowa Medical Society*, November 1968, p. 1130.

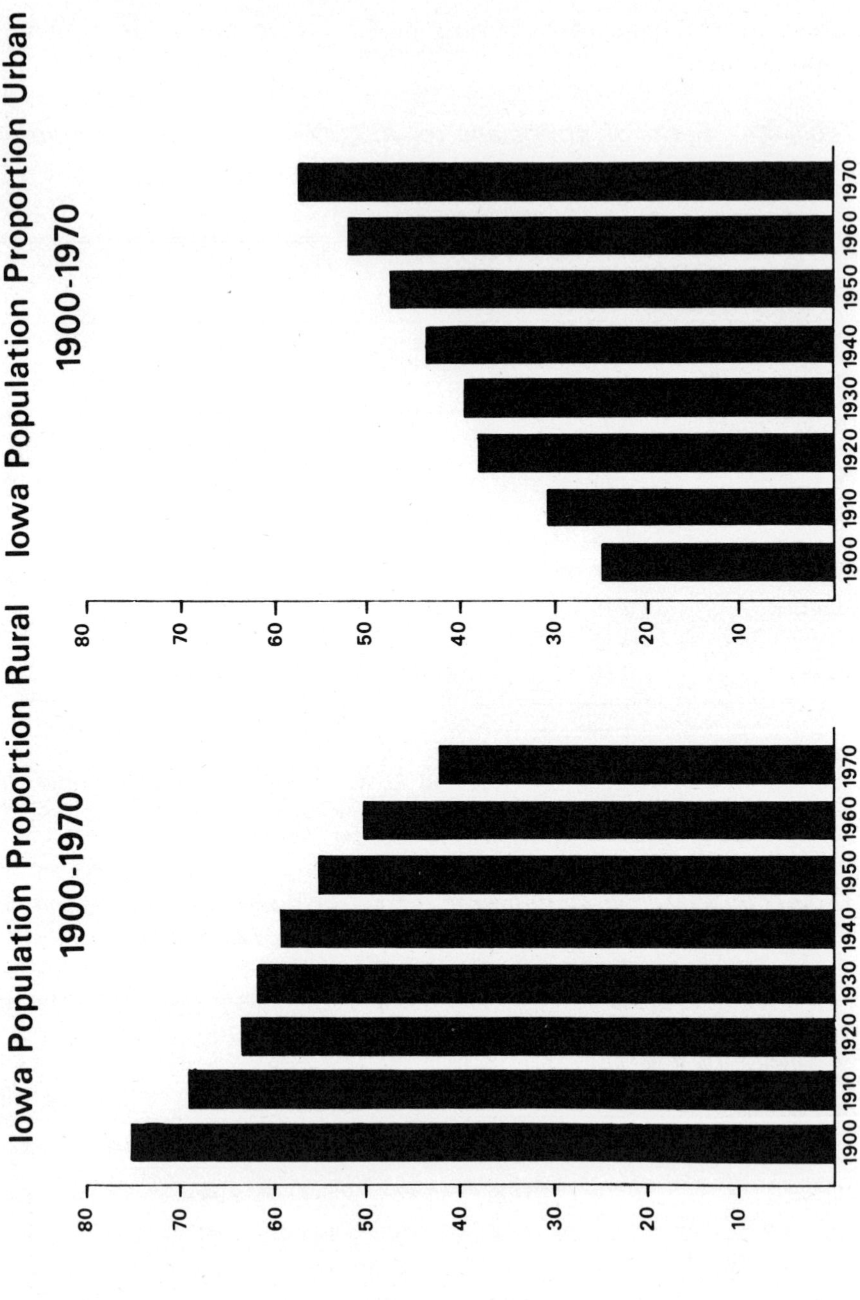

Figure 3.12. Change in Iowa urban and rural population proportions, 1900-70.

Table 3.6. Changing age structure of physicians in rural villages in Iowa by decade, 1910-1960

Population of Village During Respective Decade	*Percentage of Physicians Age 60 or Older*					
	1910	*1920*	*1930*	*1940*	*1950*	*1960*
Under 500	8	18	34	54	64	84
500–999	11	18	30	45	46	63
1000–1499	13	23	26	40	45	52
1500–2500	15	24	36	42	41	52

Source: MacQueen, op. cit., p. 1132.

MacQueen states that during the period from 1910 through 1940, there was a physician in almost every town and hamlet. Thus, this relatively ubiquitous health resource created an "expectation" on the part of (Iowa) citizens that physicians would be geographically nearby. This expectation remains, to a greater or lesser degree, *"in spite of evidence that greater mobility and modern transportation have made good medical care available to rural families."* Such "evidence" is disputed by some–particularly by the rural poor. In a recent series of hearings investigating the rural health crisis, it was concluded that most of the rural poor know where to get health care; the real difficulty is getting there. Clinics are viewed as inaccessible in terms of distance, as reflected in travel cost and time. One witness put it this way, "Tuesday you spend all day at (a) baby clinic. Thursday you take the older kids to another clinic for shots. If you need a shot for your shoulder (bursitis) you have to go to a county hospital miles away."[29]

A study of a rural county in North Carolina demonstrated a significant difference in white-non-white participation in pre-natal health care patterns.[30] This investigation indicated that "place of residence, the desire to secure care close to home, and from familiar sources, may be the most important determinants." Also, "There was a strikingly more consistent use of health department facilities in the norhtern part of the country, where physicians in private practice were scarce and the distance to hospital clinics a formidable barrier to families without cars and limited income."[31]

This lack of adequate health care is reflected in the health statistics of rural areas. Recent government studies document the relatively unhealthy status of the rural population.[32] For example, nearly seventeen percent of the rural population has some form of medical condition that limits activity, whereas the proportion of urban residents showing similar conditions is about ten percent.[33] The majority of these conditions are chronic. Of equal concern, the infant mortality rate (considered one of the most reliable indexes of the health of a population) was highest in the most rural and poverty stricken areas.[34] The Report of the President's National Advisory Commission on Rural Poverty indicated that, for the period from 1961 to 1965, the infant mortality rate in rural areas was 29.2 deaths per 1000 live births, while the total figure for the United States was 25.1 and the rate for metropolitan areas was 24.1. Rural areas tend to exhibit a higher infant mortality rate regardless of race. Among white infants born in metropolitan areas the mortality rate was 21.4 deaths per 1000 live births; while the rate for white infants in rural areas was 24.2. The mortality rate for non-white infants in metropolitan areas was 38.2 deaths per 1000 live births compared to a rate of 49.5 for non-white infants in rural areas.[35] Figure 3.13, shows the currently available infant mortality statistics. It is interesting to note that high infant mortality rates are concentrated in the Southeastern United States. It should be pointed out that this area also has the greatest percentage of black population and further, the highest concentration of lay mid-wives. Thus, it is evident that the heaviest burden of inadequate health care falls on the shoulders of the rural poor non-white. Further treatment of the white-non-white differential in health status is presented when intra-metropolitan patterns are discussed. It is interesting to note here, however, the tragically higher infant mortality rate maong the non-whites regardless of rural or metropolitan classification.

Similarly, fatality rates for accidents in rural areas are nearly four times higher than for accidents occurring in urban areas. This fact has been attributed to delays in receiving emergency treatment, due to the lack of facilities in these areas, and the time

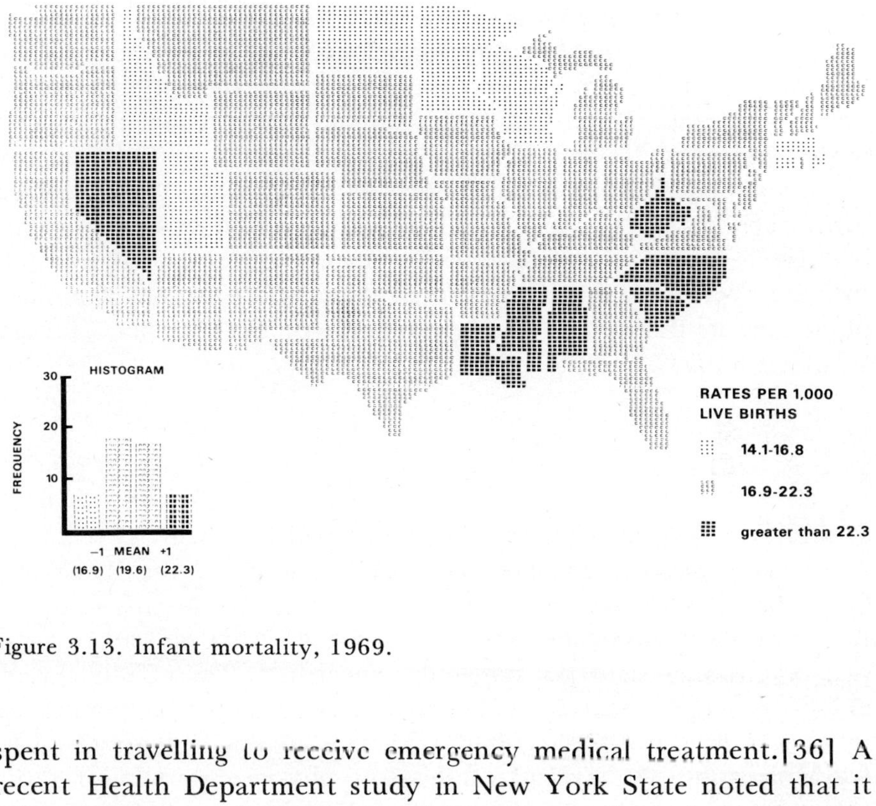

Figure 3.13. Infant mortality, 1969.

spent in travelling to receive emergency medical treatment.[36] A recent Health Department study in New York State noted that it takes an average of sixty-nine minutes for an injured or ill person to be taken in an ambulance to a hospital and to be attended by a physician.[37] It took an average of fifteen minutes from the time of an accident, a heart attack or other health crisis for an ambulance to arrive and eighteen minutes more before the patient arrived at the hospital. The report also indicated that the delay in seeing a doctor in emergency rooms in rural areas is noticeably higher than in urban areas, the average being twenty-five minutes.

Rural populations are also characterized as receiving less medical care than their urban counterparts. This is demonstrated by fewer physician visits in rural areas than in urban.[38] In some areas ninety percent of rural poor patients examined have multiple pathologies, the simultaneous occurrence of different diseases. Often, several of the diseases are in a fairly advanced stage.[39]

Intra-metropolitan Variations

In contrast to the plethora of information that exists pertaining to rural-urban differentials in physician location, there are only a few substantive studies that have concentrated on the intra-metropolitan differentials. Terris and Monk noted, almost incidentally, that physicians were leaving not only rural areas but also the "low socio-economic" areas of the cities with no prospect of replacement. This dual migration: rural to urban and inner city to suburbia has been typical of selective segments of the population and likewise typical of the physician. Evidence of depletion of primary physicians in the inner city is presented for Los Angeles, Chicago, Washington, D.C. and Cleveland.

LOS ANGELES

Within Los Angeles County, the South and Southeast Districts of the Health Department are comprised mainly of the Watts and Willowbrook sections. The combined districts contain approximately 330 private physicians. Of these, seventy-seven percent are general practitioners and the remainder specialists. The effective availability is approximately 158 physicians, a physician-population ratio of 1:3,000 or 33.3:100,000. (This is similar to the ratio cited for Mississippi.) As a result of this low physician-population ratio, the main source of primary medical care is the 3,000 bed L.A. County-University of Southern California Medical Center about twelve miles away. The complex, via an inadequate and unreliable transportation system is two hours and $1.75 away.[40] Obviously, a problem of accessibility exists for inner-city black residents.

CHICAGO

Information regarding Chicago's primary medical care delivery system is available and pertinent. The health picture of ghetto residents in Sandburg's "City of the Big Shoulders" portrayed by the infant mortality rate is indeed grim. In Cook County twenty-five infants die for each 1000 live births. However, rates based on economic status reflect that the number of infant deaths per 1000 births is 38.5 for poverty areas and 22.2 for non-poverty areas. For non-whites the rate is 43.0 versus 22.0 for whites. The number of infants dying in a non-white poverty area is 45.5 for each 1000 births. The contrast is even sharper when a neo-natal mortality rate of 60.6 for the sub-community of Kenwood A—a black ghetto—is compared with the 8.6 of neighboring white, middle-class Hyde Park.

The importance of the differential in primary health care is most evident in mortality rate for cancer of the cervix (detectable by the Pap Smear). This disease reaches a peak of 7.2 per 100,000 among black women living in poverty and only 3.0 per 100,000 among white women above the poverty level. Similarly, rates for tuberculosis and several other diseases are higher among the impoverished ghetto residents.[41]

The changing availability of physicians is clearly demonstrated for Chicago. In 1930, the all-white community of East Garfield Park had 212 physicians' offices within the community. Today there are thirteen physicians to serve the 63,000 residents of the same—but now black—neighborhood. Similarly the Kenwood-Oakland sub-community on the Southside had, in 1930, 110 physicians and 28,400 white residents. Recently (1969), there were five physicians for 45,400 Negroes. As a final example, in 1930 Woodlawn and Uptown were communities of similar ethnic composition. Thirty years later Woodlawn is approximately ninety-four percent non-white, and Uptown has a population of just over two percent non-white. In 1930, Woodlawn had 122 doctors; today it has only fourty-four, and the number of physicians in Uptown during the same period has increased from 120 to 219.[42] White-non-white differentials of physicians' locations is illustrated in Table 3.7.

It has also been documented that more than half of all "services" rendered to 285,000 welfare recipients in Chicago in 1967 were supplied by just seventy-three physicians. Medicare and Medicaid have evidently also produced a new breed of physician—the mass production specialist—who sees up to 150 patients per day and receives payment from the government of up to and beyond $100,000 a year. Of the five physicians practicing in the Kenwood-Oakland community of 45,400 residents, two were cited by the Chicago Board of Health for operating unsanitary medical facilities. In 1968, one physician received $95,729 and another received $87,643 for treating public aid recipients.[43]

Table 3.7. Average numbers of physicians and characteristics for all tracts and white and black tracts separately, Chicago, 1960

	All Tracts	*White Tracts*	*Black Tracts*
No. of Physicians	5.31	5.87	1.69
No. of G.P.'s	3.09	2.98	1.16
No. of Specialists	2.22	2.89	.53
Populations	4,524	4,591	4,332
% Commercial Area	6.89	6.57	7.59
No. of Hospital	.08	.09	.03
% 25 yrs. old or older	60.07	61.03	53.24
% H.S. Graduate Plus	31.80	32.80	24.76
% $6,000	54.88	58.83	32.09
N=	792	671	115

Source: D. Elesh and P. Schollaert, "Race and Urban Medicine: Factors Affecting the Distribution of Physicians in Chicago," *Journal of Health and Social Behavior,* 13, September 1972, p. 241.

WASHINGTON, D.C.

A similar differential in physician distribution has been documented for four quadrants of the District of Columbia (Table 3.8). Of the 1524 physicians in office-based practice, including 270 in general practice, ten percent were situated in the southeast and northeast quadrants of the city containing fifty-seven percent of the predominantly black population.

CLEVELAND

Physician emigration and avoidance of low-income, non-white areas of our cities has been demonstrated. Nevertheless, Figures 3.14 and

*Table 3.8. Ratio of office-based physicians practicing in each quadrant of the Dictrict of Columbia to percentage of population residing within each quadrant, 1969**

Quadrant	*Percent*
Southeast	0.16
Northeast	0.23
Southwest	1.00
Northwest	1.87

*Ranked from poorest to richest quadrant
Source: R. R. Huntley, "Primary Medical Care in the United States: Present Status and Future Prospects," *International Journal of Health Services*, vol. 2, no. 2, May 1972, p. 197.

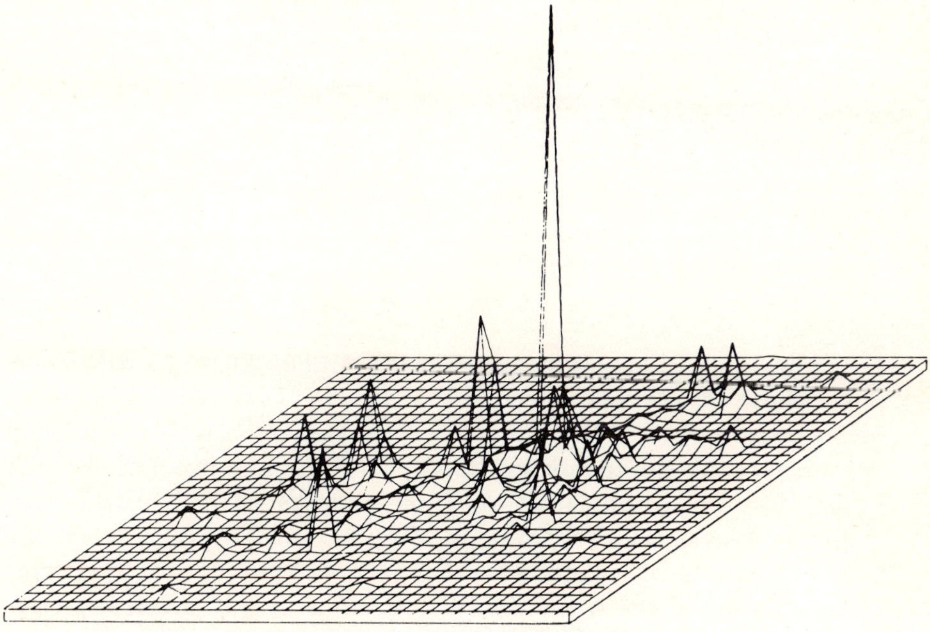

Figure 3.14. Distribution of physicians as shown by a three-dimensional model.

3.15 illustrate that in Cleveland physicians are not far removed from the non-white area. The non-white, low-income Hough area appears to be bordered on at least two sides by the highest

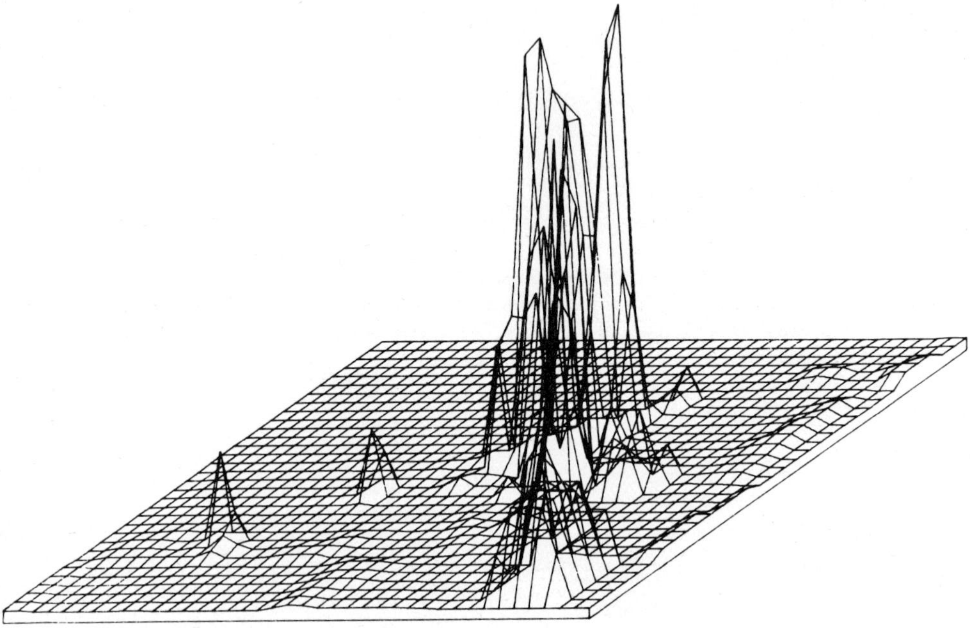

Figure 3.15. Percent distribution of non-white population as shown by a three-dimensional model.

concentrations of physicians in Cleveland. The highest peak represents those physicians with offices in the Case-Western Reserve Medical Complex. The number of physicians in this area and within a one mile radius surrounding the Center account for just under thirty-nine percent of the total number of practicing physicians in Cleveland. The second largest concentration is in the Central Business District, including 5.2 percent of all physicians and a total of eleven percent within a radius of one mile.[44] Over forty percent of all physicians have offices in close proximity to the Hough community. (It should be mentioned that a large majority of these are specialists.) A representative sample of the Cleveland Area population obtained in one study indicated that the

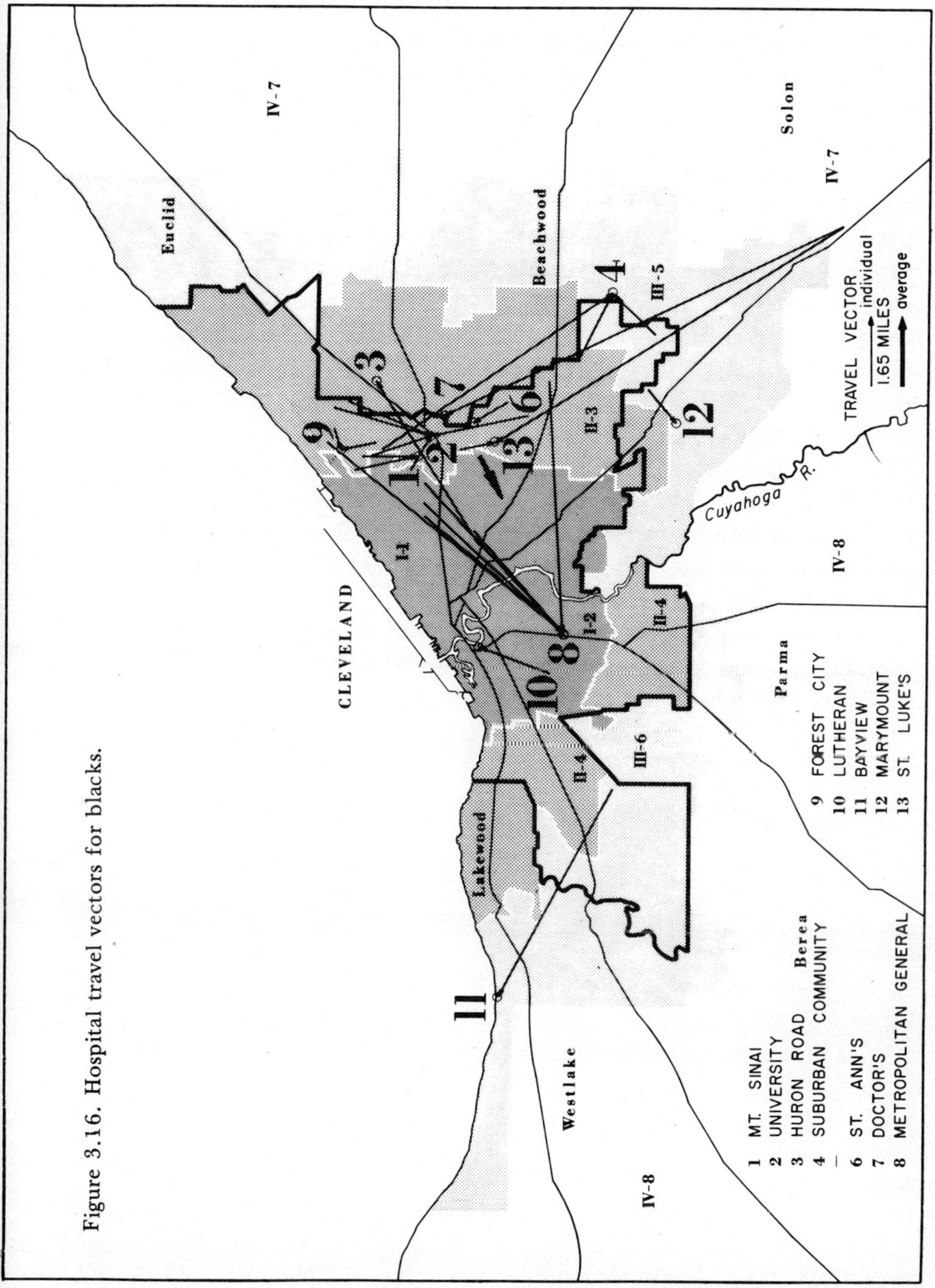

Figure 3.16. Hospital travel vectors for blacks.

average distances to the nearest as well as the second nearest physician were less for non-whites than the average distance to the nearest phvsician for any other identified group (.33 miles and .45 miles respectively). The highest peaks of physicians, though many are specialists, are almost across the street from the major black enclave.

Other than the Jewish population, the blacks are least "efficient" in their travel patterns to physicians. Over ninety-seven percent of the black population travels beyond the second nearest physician for care. Similarly, blacks on the average are only one and one-half miles from the second nearest hospital. Yet again, with the exception of the Jewish population, the non-white group has the highest percentage of patients traveling beyond these facilities.[46] As Figure 3.16 illustrates, the blacks travel across the Cuyahoga River for treatment at Metropolitan General Hospital. Likewise, similar extensive travel patterns for non-whites to Chicago's Cook County Hospital have been documented.[47] It is obvious that discrimination, of both a racial and an economic nature, plays important roles in determining the use of "health space" for a group which, in many cities, is a majority of the population.

Why are the physicians distributed as they are? What are the parameters that influence the locational decision of a physician? Answers to these questions may determine, in part, our ability to cope with the maldistribution problem.

REFERENCES CITED

[1] D. Mechanic, "Problems in the Future Organization of Medical Practice," *Law and Contemporary Problems,* 1971, p. 240.

[2] E. Ginsburg and M. Ostow, *Men, Money and Medicine:* Senate Staff Report, 1969
Mechanic, op. cit.

[3] H. K. Schonfeld, J. F. Heston, and I. S. Falk, "Numbers of Physicians Required for Primary Medical Care," *New England Journal of Medicine,* vol. 286, March 16, 1972, pp. 571-576.

[4] D. A. Clark, et. al., *Organization and Administration of Group Medical Practice,* Joint Committee of the 20th Century Fund and the Goodwill Fund, and Medical Administration Service, Inc., October 1941.

[5] J. B. Pastore, *Medical Care Program,* Report to the Committee on Future Plans of the New York Hospital and Cornell University Medical College, October 1945.

[6] J. W. Mountin, and E. H. Pennell, *Health Service Areas,* Federal Security Agency, Publication No. 305, Washington, D.C., 1949.

[7] S. Joroff and V. Navarro, "Medical Man Power: A Multivariate Analysis of the Distribution of Physicians in Urban United States," *Medical Care,* vol. IX, no. 5, September-October 1971.

[8] Ibid., p. 574.

[9] Ibid., p. 575.

[10] J. N. Haug, G. A. Roback, and B. C. Martin, *Distribution of Physicians in the United States, 1970,* A.M.A. Chicago, 1971.

[11] F. G. Dickinson, *Distribution of Physicians by Medical Service Areas; Bureau of Medical Economic Research,* A.M.A. Chicago, 1954, p. 161.

[12] R. B. Kennedy, "Milestone 300,000: Medical Progress and Doctors for All," *Journal of Mississippi Medical Association,* vol. VII, no. 6, June 1966, p. 287.

[13] M. Y. Pennell, J. E. Renshaw, "Distribution of Women Physicians, 1970," *Journal of the American Medical Women's Association,* vol. 27, no. 4, April 1972, pp. 197-203.

[14] D. Elesh and P. T. Schollaert, "Race and Urban Medicine: Factors Affecting the Distribution of Physicians in Chicago," *Journal of Health and Social Behavior,* 13 (September), 1972, p. 239.

[15] J. A. Roth, "The Treatment of the Sick," pp. 214-243 in *Poverty and Health,* ed. by John Kosa et. al., Cambridge, Harvard University Press.

[16] M. A. Haynes, "Distribution of Black Physicians in the United States, 1967," *J.A.M.A.*, vol. 210, no. 1, October 6, 1969, pp. 93-95.

[17] G. Yamamoto. "Black Phvsicians Survey," National Medical Association Foundation, 1972.

[18] M. I. Roemer, "Historical Development of the Current Crisis of Rural Medicine in the United States," *Victor Robinson Memorial Volume: Essays in History of Medicine,* ed. by S. Kagan, New York, Froeben Press, Inc., 1948, pp. 333-342, p. 335.

[19] Roemer, op. cit., p. 334;

[20] H. S. Perloff, E. S. Dunn, E. E. Lampart, and R. F. Muth, *Regions, Resources and Economic Growth,* University of Nebraska Press, 1965, p. 172.

[21] Roemer, op. cit., p. 336.
[22] A. Flexner, *Medical Education in the United States and Canada,* Report to the Carnegie Foundation for the Advancement of Teaching, Bulletin Number 4, 1910, New York, The Carnegie Foundation for the Advancement of Teaching, 1910, pp. 15-16.
[23] M. M. Davis, *Public Medical Services: A Survey of Tax Supported Medical Care in the United States,* Chicago, 1937, p. 87. (Cited in Roemer, p. 337.)
[24] J. W. Mountin, E. H. Pennell and V. Nicolav, "Location and Movement of Physicians, 1923 and 1938—Effect of Local Factors Upon Location," *Public Health Report,* 57: 1945-1953. December 18, 1942.
[25] M. Terris and M. Monk, "Recent Trends in the Distribution of Physicians in Upstate New York," *American Journal of Public Health,* May 1956, pp. 585-591.
[26] Ibid., p. 587.
[27] A more recent study is available comparing the distribution of medical and osteopathic physicians in the United States: M. Monmonier, "Comparative Geography of Medical and Osteopathic Physicians, in the United States, 1967: *Proceedings* of the Middle States Division, Association of American Geographers, vol. 6.
[28] MacQueen, vol. LVIII, no. 11, pp. 1129-1135.
[29] B. H. Alexander, "Chronic Illness—Fact of Life for the Rural Poor," *Hospitals,* vol. 43, July 1, 1969, pp. 71-74.
[30] A. D. Peters, and C. L. Chase, "Patterns of Health Care in Infancy in a Rural Southern County," *A.J.P.H.,* vol. 57, no. 3, March 1967, pp. 400-423.
[31] Ibid., p. 421.
[32] *Health Care in Rural America,* U.S. Department of Agriculture, Economic Research Service, Washington, D.C., Government Printing Office, July 1970 and *Rural Poverty in the United States,* President's National Advisory Commission of Rural Poverty, Report, Washington, D.C., Government Printing Office, May 1968.
[33] *Health Care,* op. cit.
[34] *Health Care,* op. cit., p. 3.
[35] J. A. McVeety, *Medical Care Delivery in Rural America: Development, Problems, and Selected Models of Delivery,* unpublished Master of Arts Thesis, Hospital and Health Administration, The University of Iowa, August 1971, pp. 32-33.
[36] R. M. Baker, *Emergency Rural Medicine,* paper presented at the 24th National Conference on Rural Health, Atlanta, Georgia, March 26, 1971, cited in McVeety, p. 34.
[37] Reported in *The New York Times,* Tuesday, October 10, 1972.
[38] President's National Advisory Commission, op. cit., p. 317.
[39] R. Strauss, "Poverty as an Obstacle to Health Progress in Our Rural Areas," *A.J.P.H.,* vol. 55, no. 11, November 1965, pp. 1772-1779.
[40] J. C. Norman, *Medicine in the Ghetto,* 1969, p. 75.
[41] E. L. White, "A Graphic Presentation of Age and Income Differentials in Selected Aspects of Morbidity, Disability and Utilization of Health Services," *Inquiry,* vol. V, March 1968, p. 19.
W. C. Richardson, "Poverty, Illness and Use of Health Service in the United States," *Hospital,* XLIII, July 1, 1969, p. 35.
[42] Norman, op. cit., p. 89.

[43] L. A. Ferguson, "What Has Been Accomplished in Chicago," in op. cit, Norman, p. 88-90.

[44] R. L. Bashshur, G. W. Shannon and C. A. Metzner, "Application of Three Dimensional Analogue Models to the Distribution of Medical Care Facilities," *Medical Care*, vol. 8, no. 5, September-October 1970, p. 404.

[45] R. L. Bashshur, G. L. Shannon and C. A. Metzner, "Some Ecological Differentials in the Use of Medical Services," *Health Services Research*, Spring 1971, p. 73.

[46] Bashshur et al., *Ecological Differentials*, p. 69.

[47] R. L. Morrill, R. J. Erickson and P. Rees, "Factors Influencing Distances Traveled to Hospitals," *Economic Geography*, April 1970.

Chapter IV

WHY PHYSICIANS ARE WHERE THEY ARE

What variables are most influential in the physician's decision to locate his practice? Is it his place of birth, the per capita income in prospective areas, the number of pharmacists, the number of nurses; or is it the number of available campsites or miles of beach or the percentage of Indians on reservations or some combination of factors? Each of the aforementioned variables and many more have been utilized, in widely ranging attempts, to "explain" the physician's location decision.

The bulk of the studies of why physicians settle where they do have been undertaken by economists using various regression analyses and other statistical devices. The studies attempt to incorporate a wide variety of data to provide information and, thus, to redress problems associated with the maldistribution of doctors. In some cases theoretical foreplay is attempted, but in others logic strange to most social scientists creeps into the analysis. For example, the the conclusion of one investigation demonstrating that more physicians are in high income areas than low, the following appears:

> . . . it is in all probability more advisable (economically) to spend a lot of physician time on high income executives, who presumably have a high productivity, rather than on low income unskilled workers. In this case, the observed spatial distribution of physicians may well be optimal, or perhaps there should still be more physicians in high income areas and fewer in low income areas. This approach, however, becomes very awkward when we extend it to the children of various income groups. To the extent that the children have comparable productive potentials, economic logic suggests that they should have comparable access to medical care.[1]

Now, it is a fact that in our society all children do not have comparable productive potentials; therefore, it must be assumed the authors appear to implicitly support differential access to physicians even among children. To be sure, lip service is paid to the concept of health from the social point of view—i.e., putting the same value on the health of all individuals—yet final statements indicate a low level of concern for this "uneconomic" consideration:

> . . . on the other hand there is good reason to believe that the uneveness in the distribution of physicians will diminish automatically, *in the long run,* along with the tendency toward regional equilization of per capita income.[2]

In the long run, of course, we'll all be dead.

Proliferation of explanatory variables is evident in early studies on the analysis of physician distributions.[3] For instance, physicians within Indiana reported a strong affinity to locate near hospitals and schools. In another study "community wealth" was found to be of "paramount" importance in determining the availability of physicians.[4] Along these same lines, another study noted that physicians might prefer to enter practice in or near the city in which they serve their internships. The quantity of medical facilities available—e.g., hospital beds—was also thought to have importance in selecting a location.[5]

Regional Factors

At the national level, regional variation in physician distribution has been explained as essentially a function of population or population and physician income. Benham, for example, demonstrates that the location of new physicians for the period of 1930 through 1960 correlates very highly with population growth and that the present distribution is best explained by population itself and not solely by physician compensation.[6]

Explanation of the areal variation in the distribution of physicians within the United States was of early concern to at least one geographer.[7] Smith selected four phenomena that were identified from earlier studies to explain the variation in physician location: population, income, medical facilities, and medical colleges. The assumption is made that a physician, viewed as a producer, would justify utilizing factors that determine locational patterns for producers. From the economic viewpoint, the producer's profit-making motives in regard to location will be dominant; and therefore, a physician will locate where such conditions are optimal. For this reason, Smith assumes that such industrial groups as communications, finance-insurance-real estate, utilities, and government are known factors in promoting economic stability. Such industries as construction, mining, and production of durable goods are also factors which tend to promote cyclic fluctuations. From these factors hypotheses are derived to explain the variations in physician distribution. He concludes that in 1950 the number of hospital beds, medical students, primary metal industries, public administration, and finance-insurance-real estate sectors provide a better explanation of physician distribution in the United States than does total population. Income does not, in itself, contribute significantly to the explanation. However, the general hypothesis that physicians prefer to locate in stable economic areas with adequate medical facilities is supported. This latter finding is corroborated by Sloan, who also found that physicians tend to locate in areas subject to less cyclical variations in income.[8]

In his economic analysis, Sloan examines the supply of physicians as a function of the demand for physician services, availability of surrogates for doctors (Nurses and pharmacists both purportedly affect physician income), and state support for medical education. He demonstrates that the age and income of a population have a positive impact in the supply of doctors, whereas the supply of nurses has a negative impact. More recently, Yett and Sloan, considering the problem of physician maldistribution, investigated factors that may affect the location decisions of recent medical school graduates.[9] There is evidence to support their hypothesis that physicians have considerable contact with a particular state—i.e., birthplace (B), medical school (M), internship (I), and/or residency training (R)—are more likely to establish first practices in the contact state. Further, greater influence is demonstrated to be exerted by the most recent contact. The problem is not solved, however, since other variables relating to income potential and general environmental conditions have a significant influence on physician location decisions.

Environmental variables, including climate and recreational facilities, are also listed as important determinants in location choice of Kansas medical school graduates.[10] A direct relationship between the size of the city of prior residence and the size of the city of practice has been demonstrated. In addition, a positive relationship between internship and residency training and a tendency to practice in the same state is supported. Perhaps the most important discovery, however, is that the wife is most influential in the choice of location for practice!

Current emphasis appears to be directed toward the B,M,I,R considerations as factors in the locational decision. Yet an earlier study indicates that when all such affiiliations are included, place of prior attachment and training account for less than half of the variance in physician distribution.[11] On an individual basis, the places of residency training, prior residence, internship, and medical college are ranked preferences in determinining the location of their practice. Further, Hassinger finds evidence in Missouri to support the notion that the large majority of rural physicians are born and educated in towns of less than 10,000, while physicians in metropolitan areas most probably graduated from metropolitan high schools.[12] Yett and Sloan agree that the most recent contact (residency) or place of training has the strongest influence for physician preference.

Finally, the affinity of physicians for medical facilities demonstrated earlier for Indiana is illustrated at a national level.[13] A substantially higher per capita concentration of physicians, especially specialists, are found in areas having medical training centers. While this concentration may be attributed to the attraction of technical knowledge available there, it is acknowledged that it is difficult to separate this effect from that of urban amenities.

Using principal components analysis to combine sixteen socioeconomic variables, Monmonier concludes, through multiple regression analysis, that the dominant control in the spatial variation of physicians across the United States is the combination of urbanization and high per capita income.[14] In an interesting companion study, Monmonier states that seventy percent of the U.S. variation for M.D.'s is accounted for by regional differences in income, urbanization, population growth, and education, while the proportion explained for osteopathic physicians (D.O.'s) is only thirteen percent.[15] Distance from an osteopathic college was determined to be an important locational factor for the latter. More importantly, osteopaths are apparently satisfying part of the demand for medical care. This is demonstrated by lower M.D.-population ratios than expected on the basis of socio-economic conditions in areas of high D.O. concentration.

If a conclusion is to be drawn from the analyses discussed thus far, it would be that physicians are strongly, but not profoundly, related to population and that the effect of income is ambiguous.

Inter-metropolitan Factors

A high positive correlation between per capita income and physician-population ratios is demonstrated in an inter-metropolitan analysis of counties grouped by degree of urbanization.[16] The study suggests, however, that an increase in the ratio is not due solely to changes in income but that income and environment change together, a factor that makes it impossible to separate their impacts. Nevertheless, the physician-population ratios are explained in terms of per capita incomes. The desire for leisure is apparently not a strong motivating force in physicians' choice of location. This low valuation of leisure is reflected by the fact that they tend not to reduce the length of their work week as their income increases. It is suggested that the tendency for physicians to cluster in relatively well-to-do areas without a loss in income may be the result of their ability to charge higher fees to these patients, who also seek their services more often. It is further hypothesized that the high concentration of physicians in very large cities (over 1,000,000) where the average physician income is less than that in smaller cities may be partly explained by cultural and professional advantages.

Using multivariate analysis for twenty-seven different physician-population ratios, it is shown that the best predictor of general practitioner rates is the percentage of population aged sixty-five years and over.[17] Race is not found to be significantly important as an explanatory variable. For specialists, education and "medical environment," including the existence of a medical school, were important determinants of location. Not surprisingly, the general hospital bed rate emerged as the best predictor of surgical specialty distribution.

These findings generally support those of Marden.[18] He also found education and medical environment to be more important for specialists than for general practitioners in metropolitan areas, but the most important variables for the distribution of the latter were the age and race characteristics of the population. Using population and age as a measure of the need for care, education as a measure of the ability to pay for it, the percentage of non-whites as a measure of the learned predisposition for it, and the number of hospital beds as a measure of the availability of supporting facilities, Marden accounted for between fifty-six and ninety-six percent of the variance. The amount of explained variance is dependent, however, upon the size category of the metropolitan area within which the analysis is performed. For this reason, the explained variance of physician distribution was highest for those areas over 1,000,000 and lowest for metropolitan areas under 50,000 in population.

Rural-Urban Factors

Why are physicians leaving and avoiding the rural areas? Mention was made earlier (Chapter III) of general centripetal forces, evolving about the turn of the century, that attracted physicians to the cities. These included the development of hospitals, the rise in wealth of urban residents, and an urban background of an increasing majority of medical students. Numerous studies have been conducted recently that attempt to identify specific factors contributing to physician migration from and avoidance of rural areas. Conclusions of these studies show a clear profile of the community and areas deficient in physicians. Areas with a relatively high percentage of the population engaged in agriculture, low median school years completed, low median income, low mobility, and low percentage of high school graduates are disadvantaged in attempts to attract and retain physicians.[19] These communities are often without adequate cultural and recreational resources, a factor that also contributes to the problem of retaining primary physicians.[20]

The establishment or existence of a hospital has no consistent effect on attempts to attract physicians to rural areas. A study of forty-two Georgia hospitals built under the auspices of the Hill-Burton Program (designed specifically to redress the rural-urban differential in health facilities) concluded (Table 4.1) that small communities are able to attract more physicians in proportion to

Table 4.1. Physician attraction in non-metropolitan Georgia communities by 42 Hill-Burton hospitals during the first year of operation

Type of Information	*Community Size*			
	Less than 2500	*2500-4999*	*5,000-25,000*	*All Categories*
Number of communities	12	17	13	47
Average population of community	1,436	3,535	12,033	3,566
Average number of beds in community hospital	24.4	30.4	73.0	41.8
Number of physicians attracted	17	28	48	93
Physicians attracted per community	1.33	1.70	3.69	2.21
Physicians attracted per 10,000 population	9.86	4.66	3.07	3.98
Physicians attracted per each 100 community hospital bed	5.80	5.41	5.06	5.30
Percent of communities not having hospital previously	83.3%	76.5%	23.1%	62.0%
Percent of general practitioners among physicians attracted	75.0%	50.0%	30.0%	44.8%

Source: R. C. Willaims and W. E. Uzzell, "Attracting Physicians to Smaller Communities," *Hospitals, J.A.H.A.*, vol. 34, July 16, 1960, p. 50.

the population and hospital size than were larger communities and hospitals. It was subsequently determined that the increased numbers of physicians were "permanent."[21]

A very different conclusion is reached for rural Illinois counties in which hospitals were constructed under the Hill-Burton Act. The greatest loss in terms of physician-population ratio occurred in those very same counties in which Hill-Burton facilities had been created during the ten years period of study. From 1950 to 1960 physicians were leaving at a rate 3½ times greater than the population. The decrease in physician-population ratio was greater in those counties in which Hill-Burton Hospitals were built than for those in which no hospital facilities existed in either 1950 or 1960. The assumption that more hospitals alone will attract more physicians appears to be in question.[22]

In an early comprehensive attempt to identify variables affecting the rural-urban distribution of physicians, Fein classifies reasons that doctors give for their first place of practice as "personal," "economic," or "professional."[23] As summarized by Hambleton, the determinants of the first and most important costs of investment to the new doctor are learning the market for his services in a given area and the type of patients he will be treating.[24] If the physician does not select his place of prior residence or a site nearby (and over half do not), he opts for a more urban area, where his employment makes a smaller dent in the local market and where his economic risks are therefore minimized. Further, it is assumed that if he chooses a more populous area he can rely more on information supplied by pharmacists, bankers, his medical school, and other doctors, thus reducing the costs of his search. Economic forces are operative in the selection of a particular site for physician practice, but not the tpye of place. The most important considerations for site selection seem to be the availability of housing and equipment (affecting costs of settlement), and the anticipated patient load (determining the time available for leisure activities and its price), which a minimum income guarantees. Professional reasons appear to be of a secondary significance and mostly involve distance to the closest hospital, the impact of which is also picked up in hours of patient care.[25]

Intra-Metropolitan Factors

There appears to be an inverse relationship between the scale and number of studies concerned with the distribution of doctors.

Consequently relatively few intra-metropolitan physician location studies have been undertaken. But, on the other hand, the intra-metropolitan studies as a group have evolved into some of the more comprehensive statements on physician distribution.

A study of the distribution of physicians in upper New York State illustrated the relationship between economic status and movement of physician.[26] Physicians were moving from the lower economoc sections of the city and were tending to congregate in "physician clusters." With the exception of specialists, this economic factor was apparently increasing in importance over time. The movement of physicians' offices away from the central city toward the suburbs, with an eye to high-income potential, has also been postulated for observed trends in Metropolitan Chicago.[27]

Among certain physicians, ethnicity appears to play an important role in the decision of where to practice; but, here too, the motive is expressed in economic terms. In a study investigating the relationship between ethnic groups and the practice of medicine, Lieberson concludes that the desire to maximize incomes appears to be a consideration for physicians to locate among their own ethnic groups.[28]

All of these studies cited above are couched in the familiar economic framework. However, another dimension is added in the work of Elesh and Schollaert. They raise the question of "whether controlling for constraints on supply and the three components of the demand for physicians services—ability to pay for, disposition for, and need for them—physicians are less likely to be found in black than in white areas of the city."[29] A model of the supply and demand is designed for physicians' services based upon the research of predecessors (Lieberson, Marde, etc.). Within this framework the effect of the race of the potential client population on the supply of physicians is investigated.

Basically, this model for the distribution of specialists and general practitioners within the Chicago metropolitan area is comprised of eight factors: four affecting demand (ability to pay, cultural predisposition, need, population size) and four affecting supply (availability of office space, availability of hospital services, accessibility to supporting population base, the effect of race). A summary of the partial regression coefficients obtained for the predictor equation is presented in Table 4.2.

Table 4.2. Summary of analyses of predictor model for physician distributions, Chicago, 1960

	All Physicians	*General Practioners*	*Specialists*
Coefficients in Standard Form			
Population (in 000s)	.338	.352	.209
% Commercial Area	.187	.204	.102
No. of Hospitals	.003	.068	.130
CBD	.091	.061	.197
% 25 yrs. old or older	.219	.199	.194
% H.S. Graduate Plus	.234	.214	.254
% $6,000 Plus	-.046	-.046	.063
% Black	-.070	-.081	.039
R^2C*	.391	.357	.319
N	792	792	792

*Corrected for degrees of freedom.

Source: D. Elesh and P. T. Schollaert, "Race and Urban Medicine: Factors Affecting the Distribution of Physicians in Chicago," *Journal of Health and Social Behavior,* vol. 13, September 1972, p. 242.

A negative effect obtained for race purportedly indicates that the compositional differences (income, age, education, etc.) are not an adequate explanation of physician distribution. The effect of race appears to be primarily centered among the general practitioners (–.081) as opposed to the specialists (-.039). This is reportedly due to the fact that approximately forty-six percent of the specialists are located in six tracts, one of which is both black and the site of a major medical center—a common feature of metropolitan areas.

Apparently unanticipated is the lack of evidence for the expected differences between the effects of income and education. The negative sign for income appears to fly in the face of the commonly accepted assumption that the physicians are fleeing to the suburbs in a desire to be in a close proximity to the higher income populations. The negative sign associated with income groups under $10,000 (determined later in the study) indicates that even families with moderate incomes may, in fact, have slightly less (geographic) accessibility to physicians than do high-income families.

Anticipated results are also obtained. For example, general practitioners are apparently influenced more by population than specialists (.352 vs. .209), and they are associated less with the CBD (.061 vs. .197). Equally unsurprising is the stronger association of specialists than general practitioners with hospitals (.130 versus .068), the latter being dependent more on commercial areas (.204 versus .102).

Race produces an eighteen percent difference in the number of physicians between black and white tracts. For this reason, it can be stated that physicians do avoid practice in black areas, and the avoiders are chiefly general practitioners. This effect may be obviated, [according to the authors.] by increasing the aggregate areal income to an "extremely high level." This observation suggests that raising the percentage of families with incomes of at least $10,000 by one percent would increase the number of physicians by only .029. The cost of raising the level of income for residents of these areas in terms of federal subsidies, etc., is clearly not a feasible alternative. We are again left with the suggestion that the most feasible alternative is to induce the physicians by financial means to locate in areas they now avoid; or alternatively, if it is decided that physicians' services should not be distributed in a market framework, the problem could be solved by assigning physicians to specific areas.

The distribution and process underlying change in the location of primary physicians in Boston and its suburbs is explained by a model based on the use of factors obtained through principal components analysis.[30] The factors "generated" by this method are socio-economic status, adult-employed, high non-white–low foreign-born, and housing units. With some exceptions these are assumed stable during the period of study (1940-1961). These factors are then used as imput into a model for studying change to investigate the relationship between the distribution of each type of primary physician and of social and economic population characteristics. Using linear regression analysis, estimates of the change coefficients are obtained.[31]

Change coefficients indicated that for Boston and suburban areas the early clusters of primary physicians observed in 1940 began to dissolve during the 1950s. While general practitioners decreased less in areas where there were more internists and pediatricians, the latter tended to increase in areas where the greatest decline in general practitioners occurred. Thus, the clusters of pediatricians and internists continued, but these clusters were less related to the location of general practitioners by 1960. Within the city proper, there was a net loss of one-half of the primary physicians from 1940 to 1961 (Table 4.3). Two-thirds of the general practitioners

Table 4.3. Physicians and populations in Boston by years

	1940	*1950*	*1961*
Population	770,816	801,444	997,197
General practitioners	1,196	1,076	367
per 100,000 population	155	134	52.6
Internists	231	260	258
per 100,000 population	30.0	32	37.0
Pediatricians	70	72	47
per 100,000 population	9.1	9.0	6.7
Total primary physicians	1,497	1,408	672
per 100,000 population	194.3	175.7	96.3
Total all physicians	2,983	3,388	3,499
per 100,000 population	387.0	421.5	501.9

Source: L. Robertson, "On the Intraurban Ecology of Primary Care Physicians," *Social Science and Medicine*, vol. 4, 1970, p. 231.

relative to the population were lost with only a twenty-three percent gain in internists and a slight loss in pediatricians. The net loss of primary physicians in the suburbs from 1940 to 1961 was one-third (Table 4.4). The losses are most dramatic for the central city because replacements of general practitioners are not forthcoming from the ranks of internists and pediatricians.

Table 4.4. Physicians and population in 70 towns and cities surrounding Boston by years

	1940	*1950*	*1961*
Population	1,433,305	1,594,739	1,870,028
General practitioners	1,312	1,275	761
per 100,000 population	91.6	79.1	40.7
Internists	48	110	235
per 100,000 population	3.5	6.9	12.6
Pediatricians	30	67	147
per 100,000 population	2.1	4.2	7.6

Source: Ibid.

Excluding the work of Sloan, Hambleton levels criticisms at the majority of previous efforts to explain the variable distribution of physicians.[32] He recognizes (1) the failure, in most instances, to provide a statistical test of theory of physician location and (2) the piecemeal fashion in which the question of physician location has been viewed, with few attempts made to integrate one determinant of the existing distribution with another. Credit is given for interesting facts that have been presented by other previous investigators including (1) a connection between the income and age of the population and physician compensation, (2) the negative impact of nurses on physician income, (3) the role of pharmacists, (4) location of last medical training in reducing the costs of setting up private practice, and (5) the importance of a nearby hospital in contributing to the physicians' leisure (apparently ignoring or unaware of contrasting results cited above). It is also recognized that a comprehensive model of physician location that utilizes not only data on the compensation of doctors but also proxies for the costs of consumption and human capital is still lacking.

A unique set of conclusions and recommendations are presented by Hambleton's model. For example, at the state level specialists appear to be most concerned about the use of their leisure time and only secondarily concerned about their expected compensation. Local recreational activity (measured in terms of beach front and camp grounds) is the strongest determinant. Adding one camp site with ten spaces for tents or trailers for every one hundred square miles of land area is linked to an increase in the specialist-population ratio of 4.3; adding a one acre beach per 100 square miles is related to a gain in the ratio of 2.19. The influence of determinants of physician compensation is relatively weak.[33]

The number of general practitioners in a state, on the other hand, is overwhelmingly determined by considerations of income, while costs of using leisure time to invest or consume seem to have no bearing on their decision to locate there. The advantage of previous training in the same state has an inconsequential negative effect.[34] Further it is noted that in increase of one percent in the representation in the states population of Indians on reservations increases the number of private general practitioners by 1.3 per 100,000 population.

At the county level, the costs of using leisure time were still dominant in the decision of a specialist to locate. The strongest force is the availability of a general hospital, which is believed to allow the physician more leisure time. The next most important element is the availability of locally developed recreational sites. Tennis courts serve as proxies for these, and adding ten new courts to county parks is linked to a gain in the specialist population ratio 2.7 per 100,000 people. Pharmacies and resident physicians trained per 100,000, serving as a proxy for familiarity of the future specialist with prospective job sites, round out the list of determinants.

General practitioners at the county level are most heavily influenced by the percentage of elderly, welfare support, and per capita income. Surprising, and apparently unexplainable, is the strong negative association between G.P.'s and hospitals: a decrease of 5.4 for every new hospital per 100 square miles. Apparently G.P.'s are attracted to population and regional characteristics not included in the model and negatively associated with hospitals.

At the postal zone level specialists seem to be associated with the percentage of elderly population: a one percentage point increase in the proportion of the population over age sixty-five results in a gain of 24.5 specialists per 100,000 population. An increase of one percentage point in the non-white population increases the specialists population ratio by 3.2. This "could be due to the tendency of specialists to practice in the commercial centers of cities near black neighborhoods, where interestingly, many elderly reside."[35]

At the postal zone level a $10 increase in rent apparently repels physicians at the rate of 9.2 per 100,000. The explanation given, remarkable as it seems, is that a decrease in disposable income is the primary consideration. Thus, we can expect that a decrease of $120 in a physician's average income of approximately $35,000 is to be a decisive factor in the locational decision. The presence of a new hospital in every postal zone raises the ratio by 0.7 and increasing the pharmacists by one for every 100,000 persons increases the G.P. ratio by 0.2.

Summary

What might we glean from the relative wealth of economic studies dealing with the physicians' location decision that will aid us in the solution of health care delivery problems, particularly those centered upon the question of health resource maldistribution? Alternatively, what direction for investigation is indicated by deficiencies in the previous approaches? Perhaps one major criticism that might be leveled against these spatial analyses is that the explanations are often limited to a demonstration of covariation of two or more sets of phenomena at one point in time or at several points in time, the assumption being one of time order or some other criteria forming the basis for causal inference.[36] A wide variety of variables have been noted to have an equally wide variety of impacts on physician distribution.

At the national regional level, for example, it is suggested that physicians tend to locate in the following regions: (1) those that are stable economically, (2) those possessing adequate medical facilities, and (3) the regions of most recent training contact. Other studies suggest that the place of prior attachment and training have relatively small impact on the distribution of physicians. Similar discrepancies are apparent in attempting to define the impact of income on locational decisions. In some instances, income exerts little influence on physician location decisions. The consensus of the studies appears to be that income potential and population income effects are ambiguous. The picture becomes more complex as we change ths scale of investigation. We find there is little agreement on variable impact on both an intra- and inter-scale level. Adding to this complexity is the differential impact of selected variables on different categories of physicians.

At the inter-metropolitan level, race was not a significantly important explanatory variable; however, in one intra-metropolitan investigation race explained, in some instances, eighteen percent of the variance. Moreover, the impact was greater for general practitioners than for specialists. Similarly, little agreement exists concerning the impact of leisure time. At the intra-metropolitan level, physicians generally place a low value on leisure; but at the state level, specialists appear to be most concerned about the use of their leisure time and only secondarily about their expected compensation. The impact again varies by the type of physician; general practitioners at the state level are apparently overwhelmingly influenced by considerations of income. At the county level, specialists are apparently still most interested in leisure time.

It is not surprising, though each study attempts to present some recommendations for policy, that little has been contributed to the potential solution of the maldistribution problem. We are told to spend money for camp sites, tennis courts, income subsidies for general practitioners, income subsidies for low-income populations, etc.; but it appears that most of the suggestions are not feasible and some not realistic. The greatest potential appears to be in the direction of the investigations by Sloan relating location decisions and contact with area. The primary constraint here appears to be a lack of data below the state level. We feel that the failure of the majority of studies to be of significant value is a result of their restricting economic assumptions, be they "economic man" and his profit maximization or whatever. The assumption that physicians in these spatial systems have perfect information about all opportunities and the assumption that physicians in such systems are homogeneous with regard to their utility function, so that they are all "economic men," may deprive these investigations of their potential utility. The shortcomings cited above are apparently realized by the investigators, and they acknowledge the intangibles of urban amenities and cultural and professional advantages as confounding factors.

The investigation of a physician's location decision is a most appropriate area for application of the behavioral approaches in geography. Heretofore, such studies have been limited primarily to locational decision-making studies in industrial or agricultural location and residential site selection. A primary contribution of the behavioral approach to geography has been the recognition of at least three basic decisions involved in the general want-satisfying problem: (1) a psychological decision to participate (i.e., deciding what to desire); (2) an economic decision to participate (i.e., deciding how much feasibility to desire); and (3) a geographic decision to participate.[37] It is also recognized that these decisions are not independent. The categories and amounts of things desired are determined through establishing a preference system via economic and psychological decisions. The distribution of these "desires" subsequently influences the individual. In the case of a physician, the "desires" influence the travel and the nature of the area to which he must go to obtain them.

Physicians do not behave optimally. They do not maximize utility as it is interpreted in a strict economic sense. A series of other motives must be considered in place of the wide acceptance of principles of economic rationalities. Including among the motives assumed to influence human decision making are the suggestions that (1) behavior is really sub-optimal; (2) behavior is the result of conflict between goals and uncertainty about roles; and (3) perhaps at a more general level, optimization principles should be replaced by the concept of bounded rationality.[38] It may, in fact, be the case that optimization of any one objective cannot be achieved without lower degrees of attainment for others. If this is the case then principles other than those of economic utility may be invoked in order to understand the choice of particular strategies.[39] Geographers have begun many lines of behavioral research including those dealing with decision making and choice behavior within the spatial framework. The physician's location decision, as well as those of other health personnel and health administrators, would appear both susceptible and appropriate areas into which to extend the behavioral approach in geography.

REFERENCES CITED

[1] G. V. Rimlinger, and H. B. Steele, "An Economic Interpretation of the Spatial Distribution of Physicians in the U.S.," *The Southern Economic Journal,* vol. XXX, July 1963, pp. 11-12.

[2] Ibid., p. 12.

[3] R. M. Dinkel, "Factors Underlying the Location of Physicians Within Indiana," *American Sociological Review,* XI, February 1946, pp. 16-25.

[4] J. W. Mountin, E. H. Pennell, and V. Nocolay, "Location and Movement of Physicians: 1923- and 1938- Effect of Local Factors Upon Location," *Public Health Reports*, vol. 47, December 18, 1942, p. 1946.

[5] J. W. Mountin, E. H. Pennell, and V. Nocolay, "Location and Movement of Physicians: 1923- and 1938- General Observations," *Public Health Reports*, vol. 57, September 11, 1942.

[6] L. Benham, A. Maurizi, and M. W. Reder, "Migration, Location and Remuneration of Medical Personnel: Physicians and Dentists," *Review of Economics and Statistics*, L, August 1968, pp. 332-347.

[7] S. W. Smith, "An Analysis of the Location of Physicians in the United States for the Year 1950," State University of Iowa, Ph.D. Dissertation, 1961.

[8] F. A. Sloan, *Economic Models of Physician Supply*, Ph.D. Thesis, Harvard University, Department of Economics, 1968.

[9] D. E. Yett, and F. A. Sloan, "Analysis of Migration Patterns of Recent Medical School Graduates," Health Services Research Conference on Factors in Health Manpower Performance and the Delivery of Health Care, Chicago, 9, December 1971, mimeo.

[10] E. D. Martin, et. al, "Where Graduates Go: The University of Kansas School of Medicine–A Study of the Profile of 959 Graduates and Factors Which Influenced Their Geographic Distribution," *Journal of the Kansas Medical Society*, vol. 69, no. 3, March 1968, pp. 84-89.

[11] H. G. Weiskotten, et. al., "Trends in Medical Practice–An Analysis of the Distribution and Characteristics of Medical College Graduates, 1915-1950," *Journal of Medical Education, vol. 35, no. 12, December* 1960, pp. 1071-1121.

[12] E. W. Hassinger, "Socio-ecconomic Backgrounds and Community Orientation of Rural Physicians," *University of Missouri Agricultural Experiment Station Research Bulletin*, August 1963, p. 822.

[13] J. E. Weiss, "The Effect of Medical Centers on the Distribution of Physicians in the United States," Ph.D. Dissertation, The University of Michigan, 1968.

[14] M. S. Monmonier, "Socio-economic Controls on Spatial Variations in the Physician Population," *Proceedings of the Pennsylvania Academy of Science*, vol. 46, 1972, pp. 91-93.

[15] M. S. Monmonier, "Comparative Geography of Medical and Osteopathic Physicians in the United States, 1967," *Proceedings of the Middle States Division, Association of American Geographers*, vol. 6 (forthcoming).

[16] Op. Cit. p. 11.

[17] S. Joroff, and V. Navarro, "Medical Manpower: A Multivariate Analysis of the Distribution of Physicians in Urban United States," *Medical Care*, vol. IX, no. 5, September-October 1971.

[18] P. G. Marden, "A Demographic and Ecological Analysis of the Distribution of Physicians in Metropolitan America, 1960," *The American Journal of Sociology*, vol. 72, no. 3, pp. 297-298.

[19] R. C. Parker, R. A. Rix, and T. G. Tuxill, "Social, Economic, and Demographic Factors Affecting Physician Population in Upstate New York," *N.Y.S.J.M.* 69(5), March 1, 1969, pp. 706-712.

[20] R. L. Crawford and M. M. McCormack, "Reasons Physicians Leave Primary Practice," *Journal of Medical Education*, 46(4), April 1971, pp. 263-268.

[21] R. C. Williams and W. W. Uzzell, "Attracting Physicians to Smaller Communities," *Hospitals,* 34(14), July 16, 1960, pp. 49-51.
[22] R. L. Durbin, "Do New Hospitals Attract New Doctors?" *Modern Hospital,* 100(6), June 1963, pp. 98-102.
[23] R. Fein, "Location of North Carolina G.P.'s: A Study in Physician Distribution," Ph.D. Dissertation, Johns Hopkins Unviersity, 1956.
[24] J. W. Hambleton, "Determinants of Geographic Differences in the Supply of Physicians Services," Ph.D. Dissertation, Department of Economics, University of Wisconsin, 1971.
[25] Hambleton, op. cit., p. 33.
[26] Terris and Monk, op. cit., p.
[27] P. H. Rees, "Movement and Distribution of Physicians in Metropolitan Chicago," Chicago Regional Hospital Study, *Working Paper, No. 12,* 1967.
[28] S. Lieberson, "Ethnic Groups and the Practice of Medicine," *American Sociological Review,* vol. 23, October 1958, pp. 542-549.
[29] D. Elesh and P. T. Schollaert, "Race and Urban Medicine: Factors Affecting the Distribution of Physicians in Chicago," *Journal of Health and Social Behavior,* vol. 13, September 1972, p. 237.
[30] L. S. Robertson, "On the Intraurban Ecology of Primary Case Physicians," *Social Science and Medicine,* vol. 4, 1970, pp. 227-238.
[31] J. S. Coleman, "The Mathematical Study of Change," in *Methodology in Social Research,* ed. by H. M. Blalock, Jr. and Ann B. Blalock, McGraw-Hill, New York, 1968, pp. 428-478.
[32] J. W. Hambleton, *Determinants of Geographic Differences in the Supply of Physicians Serviced,* Ph.D. Dissertation, Department of Economics, University of Wisconsin, 1971.
[33] Ibid., p. 130.
[34] Ibid., p. 143.
[35] Ibid., p.
[36] Robertson, op. cit., p. 228.
[37] R. G. Golledge, L. A. Brown and S. Williamson, "Behavioral Approaches in Geography: An Overview," *The Australian Geographer,* XII, 1, 1972, p. 62.
[38] Ibid., p. 64.
[39] Ibid., p. 64.

Chapter V

IMPACT OF GEOGRAPHIC FACTORS ON HEALTH CARE:

The Recipient

It is quite obvious that an individual's daily-activity space, or the locations that individuals utilize in their daily activities, determines the complexities of environmental factors that his system will experience. Among these factors are those that may lead directly or indirectly to disease development. This has been the traditional corner stone of medical geography. Earlier, however, a list and brief discussion of problems were presented pertaining to the classical approach in medical geography. Included in the list were factors intrinsic to the patient, factors associated with the socio-economic environment and factors related to hospital and clinic care as they affect availability and accessibility and thus the utilization of health service. As Girt and others point out, the effect of the availability and accessibility of medical services on spatial patterns of disease has been neglected by geographers.[1] Recently, the profession has also become interested in the corollary problem of locating medical facilities. Both illness and therapeutic behavior have important spatial components.

Illness and Therapeutic Behavior

The concept of illness behavior refers "to the ways in which given symptoms may be differentially perceived, evaluated, and acted (or not acted) upon, by different kinds of persons.[2] The concept as originally proposed included differential response to symptoms by reason of education, religion, class membership, occupational status (or whatever) . . . which causes some persons to make light of symptoms, shrug them off, and avoid seeking medical care and others to respond to the slightest twinges of pain or discomfort by quickly seeking medical care as it is available."[3] It has been recently hypothesized and demonstrated that with increasing distance from a health care facility an individual's sensitivity increases. He is more likely to be aware of health-threatening situations or developments when isolated in a wilderness area, for example, than he would be if living adjacent to a major university hospital. Thus, with increasing distance from a health facility awareness of health status increases. Conversely, the more distant one is from a health facility, the greater the effort necessary to obtain health care. Consequently, therapeutic behavior, "behavior relating to the decision to seek medical care once it has been recognized that a state of illness does exist,"[4] is likely to be negatively affected by distance. The desire to eliminate ill-health probably decreases with increasing distance because of the effort involved in travel and the possible deprivation of other satisfactions enjoyed during the time spent in the journey. Of course this spatial component of illness and therapeutic behavior varies with the severity of the threat or danger to health status. One would expect that consulting a doctor for less serious, uncomfortable diseases would be more critically influenced by distance than others.

Generally, research pertaining to the impact of geographical factors of recipient health care behavior is analogous to that conducted into consumer behavior. For example, Huff suggests:

> (1) consumers show a willingness to travel further distance for various goods and services as the number of such items available at various locational sources increase; (2) the anticipated cost of transportation, the time and effort involved in preparing for, as well as making the trip, and other opporutnities that must be foregone, tend to bring about a contraction in travel distances; (3) generally, consumers of higher economic status travel further for shopping purposes than consumers of lower economic levels; and (4) the greater the density of population of an area, the greater is the friction of distance, and therefore, the shorter will be the distances that consumers will travel in making their purchases.[5]

Consumer travel movements are therefore primarily a function of: (1) the relative number of particular product offerings at various locational sources; (2) the cost associated with traveling to the numerous locational sources; (3) the variations that exist among products of different types; (4) the variations among consumers of differing economic classes, and (5) the variable response to the friction of distance. Many of these concepts cited above, as well as others, have been examined as they pertain to health care delivery. Subsequent demonstration of these concepts will provide a basis from which the impact of the availability and accessibility of medical services on spatial patterns of disease may be approached.

CONCEPT OF DISTANCE*

Interest in the concept of distance between patient and provider as it related to utilization of health services may be documented for some 120 years in the published literature. However, the bulk of this material has been presented within the past forty years, and only recently have journals been established within which such articles are concentrated.[6] Therefore, an important function of this section is to present the major findings and trends of this area of interest and to provide an overview of past efforts. Research using the variable of distance has evolved from some studies based on areal concepts that deal largely with the distribution of personnel and facilities to studies that demonstrate explicit empirical relations between utilization and finally to those investigations based on systematic use of theory. Since these types of studies still coexist, a partial review of the literature may serve to call attention to the progress of current procedures for handling spatial relationships and distributions and also to current problems in relating both methodology and theory to health issues.

Many investigators interested in the problems of distribution of personnel have turned toward individual phenomena and have obtained measures of distance between patient and provider of service. This approach has the advantage of making possible a

*This section is based upon an earlier work by G. W. Shannon, R. L. Bashshur, and C. A. Metzner, "The Concept of Distance as a Factor in Accessibility and Utilization of Health Care," *Medical Care Review,* vol. 26, no. 2, February 1969, pp. 143-161.

measurement of need, or at least of utilization. Frequently, distance is measured not for individuals, but between central points of various areas, and involves the difficulties of areal correlation.

Travel time has been used as a measure of effort, with success, but this omits other phenomena related to human effort; for instance, habitual use of a road as contrasted with unfamiliarity, and whether the trip is used to accomplish a number of things so that only part of the effort need be attributed to the receipt of medical care. Travel time also varies by time of day and direction of travel in different areas, a factor that makes standardization difficult. Perceived travel time may be a better resultant measure of effort than objective clock time.

Theoretical developments in geographical analysis have occurred mainly in fields other than health care. These theories appear to be applicable to health functions and in some cases have been demonstrated. Much of this geographical theory was developed in the latter part of the nineteenth and early twentieth century.

It has long been observed that the location and social activities of people are spatially ordered. In fact, distributions can describe the spatial location of most forms of institutional behavior. This distributional pattern assumes (1) a central core that is the area of highest concentration of the phenomenon under consideration and (2) the gradual decline in the density of the phenomenon as distance from the core increases. This latter aspect has been labeled a "distance decay function" or a "gradient pattern."

The concept of gradient, of course, includes not only phenomena that diminish with increasing distance but also phenomena that increase with increasing distance from a central core. For instance, early reported incidence of juvenile delinquency, adult crime, schizophrenia, and family detachment show a distance decay.[7] On the other hand, certain other organizational variables, such as family stability and formal and informal group membership, have been shown to have a positive association with distance from the urban center.[8]

The major theoretical impetus for studies relating to the distance or gradient concept can be traced to Von Thunen.[9] Von Thunen asserted that, given an open expanse of land and a city located in the center, location of all activities would be competitively related to the city center. He demonstrated, utilizing marginal economic analysis, the attentuating effect of distance in terms of location of agricultural functions. Christaller extended this notion to tertiary activities in his central place theory.[10]

Some of the earliest attempts to deal with the effect of distance on social interaction were conducted in England[11] and Sweden.[12] The association observed between increasing distance and decreasing volume of migration proved so striking in those studies that a number of attempts were made to express this relationship in a more general, often mathematical form.[13]

The question that was generally posed for most of the previous health research reported may be stated as follows: What is the impact of geographic factors on the acquisition of various medical services? Although it is not explicitly stated in these terms, the question implicitly assumes that the specific location of services is not important in terms of the hypothesized basic relationship; that is, the effect of distance on utilization of medical services is not influenced by the particular location of these services. This assumes that any location, in the city or outside of it, is equivalent to any other location equally distant from the individual whose actions are studied. As we have seen this assumption is highly questionable. Indeed spatial location involves specific biases within an area, since these are usually defined by the cultural norms that are commonly accepted in that area. For instance, a Catholic hospital is unlikely to be built in a Jewish neighborhood, nor will a physician ordinarily locate in a "red light district" or, as we have seen, in an urban ghetto. Similarly, for a black patient residing in a ghetto the subjective economic distance increases sharply for a facility located in a white suburb and vice versa.

SELECTED MODELS OF INTERACTION

Geography has provided a certain degree of sophistication in constructing models dealing with the distance variable. The elementary interaction models developed to explain the fall-off or lapse rates have been of two kinds—models that draw heavily on physical analogues and models of a general mathematical form, which are empirical attempts to generalize detailed findings.[14] Borrowing directly from the physical sciences, geographers have applied concepts from the field of gravitational theory somewhat successfully.[15] It was suggested early, by Reilly, that movement between two centers would be proportional to the product of their populations and inversely proportional to a power of the distance separating them;[16] i.e.,

$$I_{ij} = \frac{P_i P_j}{D_{ij}^{\ b}} \tag{1}$$

where I_{ij} = the interaction between cities i and j,
P_i = population of city i,
P_j = population of city j,
D_{ij} = distance between cities i and j,
b = empirically estimated exponent.

The above formulation represents the general expression for the "gravity" or "interaction" model. Of particular interest to us here is the value of the exponent, since the higher it is, the greater is the "friction" of distance in interaction; that is, the downward slope of the curve is steeper. It might thus be expected that the exponent would be greater for travel to general practitioners than to specialists, since people go farther to specialists.

Migration studies have also provided a great deal of empirical information concerning the varying impact of distance upon social interaction and movement. Generally, the interaction level (in terms of migrants, journeys to various facilities, informal associations, etc.), as related to the distance of these journeys, has been expressed in a number of ways—as normal, log-normal, quadratic, and Pareto functions. It has been demonstrated, for example, that the numbers of immigrants to a Scandinavian town can be represented by a Pareto-type formula:[17]

$$M = aD^{-b} = \frac{a}{D^b} \tag{2}$$

where M is the number of migrants, D is the distance from the place of original residence, and a and b are constants. This function is a simplification of the formula for the "gravity" model given above. Whatever the type of expression utilized, interest centers around the value of the exponent b. Again low values of b indicate relative ease or willingness to movement with more restricted movement or resistance to movement indicated by a corresponding increase in the value of b.

The transfer of these concepts to health care delivery is somewhat obvious. It is only necessary to substitute "patients" for "migrants" or percent of patients who travel to seek health care for "interaction level" and distance travelled to a medical facility for "distance" in order to examine the relationships between these variables. This has been done in several instances as will be shown in the subsequent section.

Distance in Health Care Delivery

The earliest reported application of distance in health care research (with important exceptions as early as 1852 and 1879 discussed in a later section) appears to be by Lively and Beck in 1927.[18] They noted the tendency for utilization of physician services to decrease with increasing distance of place of residence from the physician. However, studying the effect of distance was somewhat incidental to the main purpose of their research.

Various publications of the Committee on the Costs of Medical Care document the unequal distribution of health personnel and facilities relative to population (physicians and hospital beds per person and per 100,000 persons) for different areal units (sections of the United States, states, and counties).[19] Since it was found that, in general, physicians (and other personnel and facilities) were most numerous relative to population in urban centers where distances were less, it could be concluded that rural people would have greater difficulty in obtaining services than urban people. In fact, the rural population would be doubly disadvantaged by having fewer available physicians (or more competition for services of a given physician) and by having to travel greater distances. Distance was not considered explicitly, and the above argument was considered sufficient to establish the existence of a problem.[20]

During the 1930s several studies followed that dealt more directly with the impact of distance on health care utilization.[21] Among the findings of this period were (1) that patients in rural areas travel between eight and ten miles to see a physician, (2) that persons residing in rural areas travel longer distances to see a physician than persons in urban areas, and (3) that the "decay function" of health care utilization was in one instance not directly associated with either an increase or a decrease in rate of illness.

An important landmark in ecological research realted to health care was published in 1939 by Faris and Dunham. The study that deals with mental illness, is worth noting in two ways:

> (1) It was the first large scale study in health care which utilized a totally ecological frame of reference; that is, the purpose of the analysis was to determine the spatial distribution of the phenomenon, not relationships to demographic or social structural variables such as income or status. . . .
>
> (2) The findings were consistent with the noted trends and further "confirmed" the applicability of geographical and ecological theory to problems of medical care in general. A gradient outward from the central area was found for schizophrenia which paralleled the gradient of social disorganization, delinquency, and like phenomena (of course confounding factors were not included, such as unreported treatment rates with increasing incomes.[22]

The enactment of the Hospital Survey and Construction (Hill-Burton) Act of 1946 was the first national expression of the need for planning hospitals and related health facilities. The major purpose of this legislation was to assist states to provide "adequate hospital, clinic, and similar services to all their people." This was to be accomplished in two phases. The first phase called for the survey of existing facilities and the development of a "comprehensive plan" setting forth the states' most pressing needs. In the second phase, Federal assistance was to be provided in the construction of hospitals, public health centers, and related facilities.[23]

This legislation, particularly the part calling for the survey of existing medical facilities, stimulated interest in their spatial distribution, and subsequent analysis focused on the distance parameter. At the time that the Hill-Burton legislation was enacted, however, problems related to the geographical distribution of medical facilities in urban centers were not considered the most pressing. Hill-Burton mechanisms were directed primarily at non-urban areas, as at that time the need there was considered the greatest.[24]

Studies were initiated to investigate where the rural populations were obtaining their health care and how well the health needs of this segment of society were being met.[25] In brief, investigations of the distribution and utilization of physicians and other medical services by the populace were common to the decade following the enactment of the Hill-Burton legislation.[26]

A study by Jehlik and McNamara was probably one of the first primarily concerned with the relationship of distance to differential utilization of various health personnel and facilities. Their purpose was to "test the hypothesis that the distance farm people reside from certain health personnel and facilities is related inversely to the use they make of such personnel and facilities, and positively related to the incidence of bed illness at home among rural and semirural populations. The main findings of this research revealed the importance of distance in explaining the patterns of health care utilization by persons living on farms. The results show that families living at greater distances from physicians tend to limit their visits largely to curative rather than preventive purposes. Further, it was concluded that as the distance that farm families reside from a physician increases, the incidence of bed illness at home also increases. It was not suggested that an increase in distance was solely associated with increase in illness, but that it was one of several factors involved—among them the socioeconomic status of the families.

Several studies have failed to support the widely reported findings that utilization declines with increasing distance from the source of care.[28] In addition to possible methodological difficulties a relatively ubiquitous distribution of resources may have contributed to at least one of these findings. For example, Altman observed a decrease in the utilization of urban-centered specialists but suggested that the lack of a significant correlation between distance and use of general physicians in western Pennsylvania could reflect the relatively large ratio of general practitioners to population and their even distribution.

In another study, Hoffer noted no relationship between distance and the number of office calls and home visits per person in areas classified as metropolitan, urban. village, and open country. However, "unmet need," indicated by one or more untreated symptoms, was positively associated with increasing distance of residence from the nearest town having a physician. The preponderance of studies, including the more recent ones, continue to substantiate the inverse relationship between the distance to a physician and utilization.

Jehlik and McNamara noted that physician consultations decrease with increasing distance from the physician and that the incidence of bed illness at home increases. This conclusion is supported by research conducted in Finland.[29] In 1964, a nationwide survey concerning the utilization of medical services and effects of the newly introduced sickness insurance scheme upon the utilization of these services was initiated. Since services rendered by physicians are important to health care, a substantial effort was directed toward an analysis of the relationship between distance and physician consultations, as well as the corollary problem of distance from physician and illness. Standardized in respect to sickness days, the average number of consultations with a physician shows a regular decrease with increasing distance.[30] The major findings are presented here:

> On average, persons living no farther than three kilometers away from the nearest physician consulted a physician about 50 per cent more frequently than did persons living at least twenty kilometers away. Both for chronically sick and for others, utilization of physician's services decreases with equal consistency with increasing distance. The difference between the extreme classes of distance is statistically significant for both groups . . . the influence of distance on the number of consultations with a physician decreases consistently with increasing distance. Utilization of physician's services thus appears to depend on distance to nearest physician and more distinctly the greater the need for medical care.[31]

Distance to the nearest physician correlated with morbidity; and with increasing distance, the relative proportion of respondents who had been sick increased. The proportion of chronically ill persons also increased considerably with increasing distance to the nearest physician. Finally, the average number of consultations with a physician generally decreases with increasing distance. Again, as in the study by Jehlik and McNamara, other socioeconomic variables are important; but the effect of the distance variables(s) is evident and substantial.

In Newfoundland, Canada, the primary source of general medical care is provided free at a series of sponsored "cottage hospitals." For a rural environment in this province, the spatial interaction component of illness and therapeutic behavior has been demonstrated. Using scores from a series of questions measuring the degree of sensitivity to ill health and its treatment, a tendency for increasing sensitivity with increasing distance of a settlement from a hospital is demonstrated.[32]

From a list of eleven diagnoses, it was found that only four diseases (acute bronchitis, acute cystitis, normal pregnancy, and sprains and strains) showed no significant variation in consultation between the settlements. The distance trends for selected examples of other diseases are presented in Figure 5.1.

The negative exponential decline relationship (Figure 5.1a) is probably indicative of the spatial interaction components relative to illness and therapeutic behavior. The illness behavior is consistently of less importance than the retarding effect of the effort involved in travelling to a doctor. The positive relationship (Figure 5.1b) indicates that the amount of effort required for consultation behavior is perhaps outweighed by illness behavior until approximately ten miles from a doctor. The third curve (Figure 5.1c)

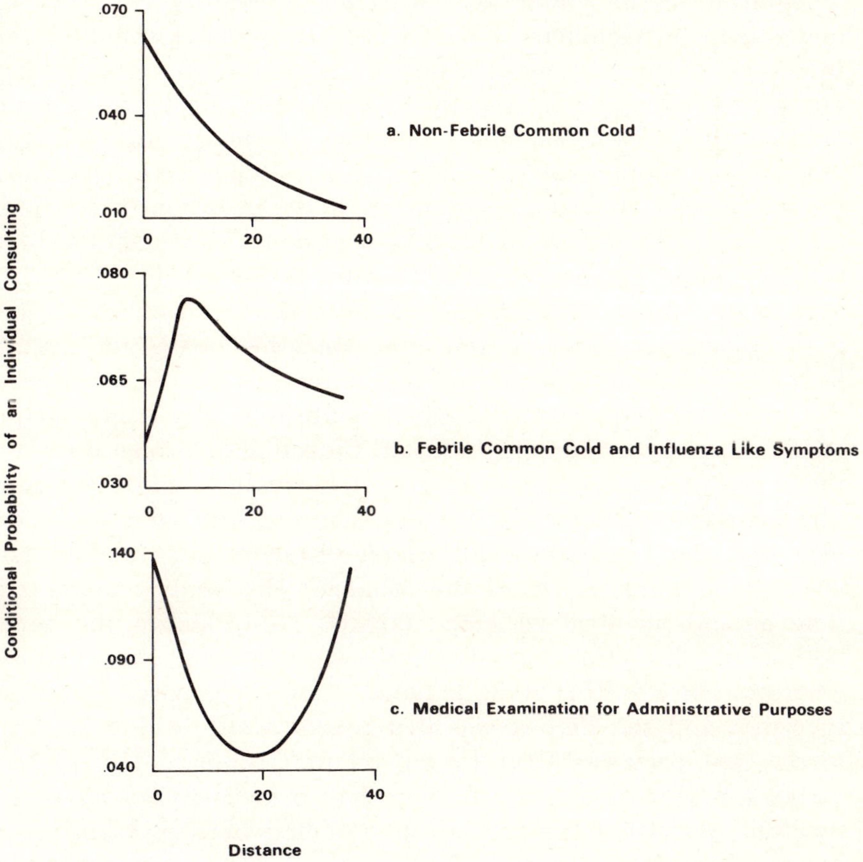

Figure 5.1. Conditional probability of an individual consulting.
Source: J. Girt, "The Location of Medical Services and Disease Ecology—Some Conclusions on the Effect of Distance on Medical Consultation in a Rural Environment."

probably reflects the availability of a physician at a weekly clinic ten miles away for the two most distant settlements.

It is obvious that the optimum location of a facility will vary with the disease. And Girt suggests this leads to a broader, more philosophical question in health planning: "Who is going to decide that more consideration should be given to maximizing consultations for one disease as opposed to another?" The fact that more people consult for common colds than for respiratory tuberculosis does not necessarily mean that more weight should be attached to finding a location closer to the optimum for colds than for tuberculosis.[33]

Applications of gravity analysis, cited previously, have also been undertaken by members of the Chicago Regional Hospital Program. It is one of the foremost planning operations in terms of geography involvement and, hopefully, a successful prototype for more rational health care planning. Evolution of gravity analysis may be linked to a monograph by Ciocco and Altman.[34] They tested the hypothesis that the relationship between distance to a physician and the frequency of visits is negatively associated. Although this is quite similar to the hypothesis tested by Jehlik and McNamara, the sophisticated treatment of the distance factor is quite different. Previous research concerned with the distance factor in medical care organization treated the measurement of distance and frequency of contact wihtout regard to the purpose of the visit or to type of physician. Ciocco and Altman noted that the patient-physician frequency is relatively high under five miles. The mathematical form ($y = a/x^b$) that was utilized expressed the idea that the frequency with which distances are travelled varies inversely as some power of the distance. This study represents the first atempt in medical care research to formalize the general notion of the effect of distance on frequency of contact. In addition, the resulting slope exponents were compared by medical specialty, and the finding was that people were "willing" to travel further to specialists than to general practitioners. This probably marks the first time that distance had been analyzed by type of medical specialty (although distinction had been previously made between medical services). Furthermore, this study introduced intra-urban in addition to rural-urban travel patterns.

Morrill and Earickson examine patient travel behavior based on hospital variation and discover, not surprisingly, that those hospitals providing the greater range of specialties "draw more patients from greater distances than do those offering a lesser range."[45] That is, the slope of the decay function in travel distance is greater for small than for large hospitals. They also found, as have others, that race, religion, and income operate to influence patient travel behavior.[36] Thus the travel behavior of blacks to distant hospitals is interpreted as a reflection of discriminatory policies relating to race and income. One the other hand, the "inefficiency" in travel behavior of certain religious groups is viewed as a distortion of distance relating to perceived desirability to seek treatment at the hospital of the denomination of their choice. They also propose that patient reaction to distance is one of "indifference up to approximately two miles." That is, there is little difference to a patient if the physician location is less than two miles from their residence; beyond two miles, however, "attractiveness" delines precipitously.[37]

Two general types of mathematical functions have been utilized in the study of the relationship between distance and the use of Chicago hospitals. Utilizing hospital admissions data, Morrill and Earickson tested two functions for "best fit." They used a power function, similar to that used by Altman presented earlier, of the general form

$$I_{ij} = \frac{a}{d_{ij}^{\,b}} , \tag{3}$$

,

and an exponential function of the general form

$$I_{ij} = \frac{a}{e^{b}\, d_{ij}} , \tag{4}$$

where, I = the number of patients from area i using a hospital in j area
d_{ij} = the distance from area i (centroid) to hospital j
b = the slope of the distance decay function
a = a constant
e = the base of natural logarithms, 2.7183.

They observed that generally, but not exclusively, the number of hospital admissions per unit area was best described by the exponential function, "although the power function did not do badly."[38] Similar results were obtained by Schultz for patient travel behavior in both fee-for-service and prepaid medical care situations. The "use of exponential as contrasted with power functions results in better prediction of actual patient spatial behavior, although the magnitude of improved prediction is moderate at best."[39]

Models of Physician-Patient Relationships

There has been a great deal of activity centered about the construction of models to replicate and predict physician and hospital use. Much of the work of the "Chicago School" involves minimizing distance for physician and patient travel through the use of gravity-interactance and potential models based on information obtained for patient behavior, hospital and physician location, etc.[40] These models attempt to replicate the use of the system. This is identified as a first requirement. The use of these models must recognize a degree of irrationality or uncertainty, and especially indeterminancy, particularly when patients are confronted with a decision between approximately equally good choices.[41] Models of physician-patient relationships must also accommodate experiment: first, to discern what models of behavior better characterize actual decision making; and second, to test the effects of possible changes in behavior or outside constraints. Finally, "the model must be able to evaluate the adequacy of the system and to prescribe changes that will raise the level of satisfaction of patients, physicians, and hospitals."[42]

Models have been constructed using various optimizing principles of spatial, social, and economic behavior. While much of the variation in behavior has been explained, these models have "come up short" in satisfying some of the above requirements. Gravity-interactance models have been satisfactory in describing the use of the system on an aggregate level. Distance-minimizing transport models are criticized for failing to allow sufficient flexibility in behavior, although they are useful in identifying groups of patients who are poorly served and hospitals that are poorly located.[43] In most cases the distance used has been linear, or some approximation, a factor that further limits the utility of the models as discussed earlier. Morrill and Earickson have constructed a simulation model that attempts to remedy the deficiencies of earlier models and meet the requirements listed above. Nevertheless, they too emphasize a reduction in patient travel as the goal of the model and express dissatisfaction with this and with the lack of emphasis on institutional viability and quality.[44] Lengthy discussion of these and other models is beyond the scope of this book, and the reader is referred to the specific studies for further details. It is appropriate, however, to briefly describe a representative model.

We have selected for presentation the HEAlth-care Delivery Simulator for Urban Population (HEADSUP) model;[45] This is a "generalized stochastic computer simulation for primary health care delivery in an urban setting" that incorporates many previous research findings.

The HEADSUP simulation model is structured upon three basic elements: patients, facilities, and services. Patients are individuals defined by: (1) their geographic location, (2) their type of need (emergency, non-emergency, referral, etc.), and (3) the health services demanded (emergency, laboratory, etc.). The physical health facilities are the basic sources of care to which the patients are allocated (Figure 5.2) according to a gravity function of the general form similar to that discussed earlier:

$$Pij = (Nj)(Dij)(Hij)(Ki) \quad (5)$$

where

$$Ki = \left[\sum_{j=1}^{N} (Nj)(Dij)(Hij) \right]^{-1} \text{ and} \quad (6)$$

$$Dij = Be^{-aTij} \quad \text{and} \quad (7)$$

$$\sum_{j=1}^{N} Pij = 1 \quad (8)$$

where Pij = probability of patient i going to facility j
Nj = number of services offered at facility j
Dij = travel time decay function
Hij = habit factor of patient i for facility j*

*The habit factor is used as a surrogate for race and religion because they are extremely difficult to measure.[46]

Tij = travel time for patient i to facility j
B = empirically derived constant
a = empirically derived travel time decay rate constant.

Each individual, thus allocated to a facility, is then passed through a "patient-facility processing module" (Figure 5.2) that

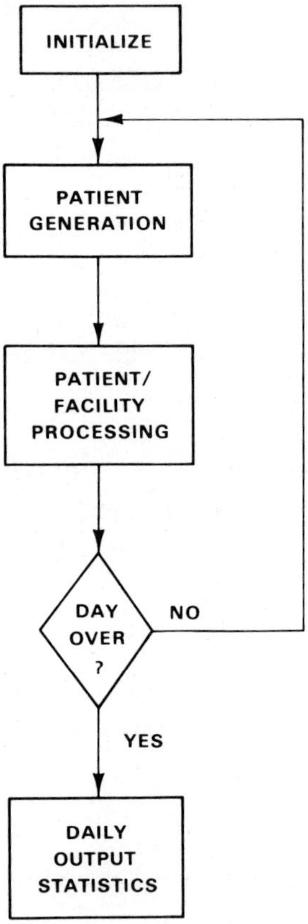

Figure 5.2. General simulation flow.

incorporates availability of service, referrals within and between facilities, and service sequence. Once the maximum feasible number of patients arriving at a facility is processed (Day Over Module, Figure 5.2), the simulator proceeds to the last module.

The final module is termed "Output Statistics" and consists of (1) level of service and (2) delivery system effectiveness. The former is measured by (a) expected facility (including travel and waiting) time for a single episode of care and (b) the expected elapse time for a single episode of care, and (c) the number of complete episodes of care. The latter consists primarily of expected patient queue time and percent utilization.

There are those, however, who question the capabilities of this type of model to deliver the design of a new delivery system. It is evident from Girt's study, for example, that distance has both a negative and positive effect on consulting behavior. If this is true then distance decay and gravity models may be inappropriate measures of the effect of distance on consulting behavior.[47] In addition, Girt suggests that "since distance does affect consultation, linear programming solutions to the location of medical facilities [48] are not appropriate since it assumes that spatial behavior does not vary with distance, only the effect involved does."[49]

Others are attempting to elaborate on this patient behavior—attempting to measure through survey research the impact of such "difficult-to-determine" variables as race and income, particularly as it affects utilization.[50] One basic structural equation presented recently takes the following regression form:

(9) $$U = f(E, P, A, H, X) + e$$

where U = utilization of various services reported by individual interviewer

E = Enabling factors; e.g., health insurance, family size, occupation etc.

P = predisposing factors; e.g., attitudes of individual toward health care, services, and physicians; health values; illness and therapeutic behavior; use of services

A = Accessibility factors; e.g., distance and/or time of individual firm facility; appointment delay time; waiting times, etc.

H = perceived health level of individual and/or family

X = individual and area-wide exogenous variables (age, sex, family size, race, location)

e = residual error term.[51]

A better understanding of the relative explanatory power of the behavioral or predisposing variables, the enabling variables, and health level indicative of health utilization is essential. To quote Gross:

> How else can health policy analysts quantitatively demonstrate the relative effectiveness of health education programs versus neighborhood health clinics as mechanisms for changing either existing health service utilization patterns and/or existing health level differentials?[52]

This we feel is a crucial question.

REFERENCES CITED

[1] J. L. Girt, "The Location of Medical Services and Disease Ecology—some Conclusions on the Effect of Distance on Medical Consultations in a Rural Environment," mimeo, 1971, p. 1.
[2] D. Mechanic and E. H. Volkhart, "Illness Behavior and Medical Diagnosis," *Journal of Health and Human Behavior,* vol. 1, 1962, pp. 86-92.
[3] Ibid., p. 87.
[4] J. L. Girt, "Distance and Patterns of Revealed Ill-Health in a Spatially-Dispersed Population: The Problem of Ascertaining Optimal Locations for general Medical Facilities," Paper presented to International Geographical Unions Commission on Medical Geography, Guelph, Ontario, 1972, pp. 2-4.
[5] David L. Huff, "Ecological Characteristics of Consumer Behavior," *Papers and Proceedings of the Research Science Association,* vol. 7, 1961.
[6] *Health Services Research, International Journal of Health Services, Health and Social Behavior, etc.*
[7] L. Wirth, *The Ghetto,* C. Shaw and H. McKay, *Juvenile Delinquency and Urban Areas*; H. Sorbaugh, *The Gold Coast and the Slum*; F. Thrasher, *The Gang,* University of Chicato Press, Chicago, 1928, 1942, 1944, 1927. R. Faris and W. Dunham, *Mental Disorders in Urban Areas,* Chicago, 1939; new edition, Hafner Publishing Col. Inc., New York, 1960.
[8] R. V. Smith, R. L. Bashshur, S. E. Flory and G. W. Shannon, *Community Support for the Public Schools in a Large Metropolitan Area,* Final Report, Project No. 2557, U.S. Department of Health Education and Welfare, May 1968.
[9] J. H. Von Thunen, *Der Isolierte Statt in Beziehung Auf Landwirtschaft,* Hamburg, 1875.
[10] W. Christaller, *Central Places in Southern Germany,* (trans. C. W. Baskin), Englewood Cliffs, New Jersey, 1966, Original German Edition, 1933.
[11] E. G. Ravenstein, "The Laws of Migration," *Journal of Royal Statistical Society,* vol. 48, 1885, pp. 167-235.

[12] T. Anderson, *Den inre omflyttninge,* Norland Malmo, 1897, in Peter Haggett, *Locational Analysis in Human Geography,* St. Martin Press, 1966, New York, p. 33.

[13] G. Olsson, *Distance and Human Interaction,* Regional Science Institute, Philadelphia, 1965.

[14] P. Haggett, *Locational Analysis in Human Geography,* 1966, p. 35.

[15] Difficulties involved in the application of physical theory to human behavior are not our major concern here. They are discussed by: D. Harvey, "Models of the Evolution of Spatial Patterns in Human Geography," Chapter 14, in R. V. Chorley, ed. by P. Haggett, *Models in Geography,* Methuen, 1967, and D. Harvey, *Explanation in Geography,* St. Martin's Press, New York, 1970, pp. 146-161.

[16] W. J. Reilly, *The Law of Retail Gravitation,* New York, 1931.

[17] T. Hagerstrand, "Migration and Area: Survey of a Sample of Swedish Migration Fields, and Hypothetical Considerations on Their Genesis," Land Studies in Geography, Series B, *Human Geography,* vol. 13, pp. 22-158.

[18] C. E. Lively and P. G. Beck, "The Rural Health Facilities of Ross County, Ohio," Ohio AES Bulletin 412, October 1927, pp. 45-46.

[19] Most of this information is detailed in Publication No. 3 of the CCMC. A. Peebles, "A Survey of Statistical Data on Medical Facilities in the United States: A Compilation of Existing Material. Summary statements are given for hospitals on p. 8 and for physicians and other personnel on p. 20. Additional material is given for hospitals on p. 37 and in Appendix 10 and for physicians in Appendix 2.

[20] The CCMC summary volume, No. 28: Committee on the Costs of Medical Care, Medical Care for the American People, the Committee, Washington, D.C., 1932, contains, in addition to summary statements, a map of Toombs Co., Ga. (Fig. 15, p. 107), giving travel distances and frequencies of use for hospitals in 1930.

[21] I. C. Wilson and W. H. Metzler, "Sickness and Medical Care in an Ozark Area in Arkansas," *Arkansas AES Bulletin 353,* Fayetteville, April 1938, pp. 37-38.
T. C. McCormick, "Rural Social Organization in South Central Arkansas," *Arkansas AES Bulletin 313,* Fayetteville, December 1934, p. 29.

[22] Faris and Dunham, op. cit., 1939.

[23] U.S. Public Health Service, "Areawide Planning for Hospitals and Related Health Facilities," PHS Publication No. 855, U.S. Government Printing Office, Washington, D.C., July 1961, p. 12.

[24] Ibid., pp. 12-13.

[25] C. Hoffer and J. F. Thaden, "Distribution of Doctors of Medicine and Osteopaths in Michigan Communities," Michigan State College, *AES Department of Sociology and Anthropology and Social Research Service, Special Bulletin 370,* June 1951.

[26] J. F. Thaden and R. Fein, "Studies on Physician Supply and Distribution," *American Journal of Public Health,* vol. 44, No. 5, May 1954, pp. 615-624.
R. L. McNamara and E. Hassinger, "The Pattern of Medical Services for Incorporated Places of 500-or-More Population in Missouri, 1950," *Rural Sociology,* vol. 21, 1956, pp. 175-177.
W. G. Mather, "The Use of Health Services in Two Southern Pennsyl-

vania Communities," *Pennsylvania AES Bulletin*, July 1948, p. 504.
M. Terris and M. A. Monk, "Recent Trends in the Distribution of Physicians in Upstate New York," *American Journal of Public Health*, vol. 46, April 1956, pp. 585-591.
[27] P. J. Jehlik and R. L. McNamara, "The Relation of Distance to the Differential Use of Certain Health Personnel and Facilities and to the Extent of Bed Illness," *Rural Sociology*, vol. 17, 1952, pp. 261-265.
[28] A. Ciocco and I. Altman, "Medical Service Areas and Distances Travelled for Physician Care in Western Pennsylvania," U.S. Public Health Service, PAS Monograph No. 19, 1954. And also see reference no. 25.
[29] T. Purola, E. Kalimo, K. Sievers and K. Nyman, *The Utilization of the Medical Services and Its Relationship to Morbidity, Health Resources and Social Factors*, Research Institute for Social Security, Helsinki, 1968.
[30] Ibid., p. 151.
[31] Ibid., p. 51.
[32] J. L. Girt, "The Location of Medical Services," p. 5.
[33] Ibid., p. 8.
[34] Ciocco and Altman, 1954.
[35] R. L. Morrill and R. J. Earickson, "Hospital Variation and Patient Travel Distances," *Inquiry*, no. 5, 1968, pp. 26-34.
[36] R. L. Bashshur, G. W. Shannon and C. A. Metzner, "Some Ecological Differentials in the Use of Medical Services," *Health Services Research*, Spring 1971, pp. 61-75.
R. L. Morrill, R. J. Earickson and P. Rees, "Factors Influencing Distances Travelled to Hospitals," *Economic Geography*, vol. 46, 1970, pp. 161-171.
[37] R. L. Morrill and R. J. Earickson, "Locational Efficiency of Chicago Hospitals: An Experimental Model," *Health Services Research*, Summer 1969, p. 131.
[38] Morrill and Earickson, "Hospital Variation," pp. 32-33.
[39] R. R. Schultz, "The Patient-Physician Spatial Relationship," Paper presented at the 69th Annual Meeting, Association of American Geographers, Atlanta, Georgia, April 15-18, 1973, p. 14.
[40] R. R. Schultz, "The Locational Behavior of Physician Establishments: An Analysis of Growth and Change in Physician Supply in the Seattle Metropolitan Area, 1950-1970," Ph.D. Dissertation, University of Washington, 1971.
R. J. Earickson, *The Spatial Behavior of Hospital Patients*, Research Paper No. 124, The University of Chicago, Department of Geography, 1970.
G. F. Pyle, *Heart Disease, Cancer and Stroke in Chicago*, Research Paper No. 134, The University of Chicago, Department of Geography, 1971.
R. L. Morrill and R. J. Earickson, "Locational Efficiency of Chicago Hospitals."
[41] Ibid., p. 129.
[42] Ibid.
[43] Ibid.
[44] Ibid., p. 140.
[45] M. A. Baum, *Primary Health Care Delivery Simulator*, Mitre Corporation, November 1971.
[46] Ibid., p. 10.

[47] Girt, "Location of Medical Services."
[48] This was suggested by P. Gould and T. R. Reinbach, "An Approach to the Geographic Assignment of Hospital Services," *Tijdschrift von Economische en Sociale Geografie*, vol. 57, 1966, pp. 203-206.
[49] Girt, pp. 8-9.
[50] P. Gross, "Economics of Health Facility Location," *International Journal of Health Services*, vol. 2, no. 1, February 1972, pp. 63-84.
[51] Ibid., p. 75
[52] Ibid., p. 75.

Chapter VI

JARVIS' LAW:

Impact of Geographic Factors on Mental Illness

This chapter is an extension of the discussion concerning the impact of geographic factors on health care for the recipient and is devoted to the evolution of a concept. The origin of this concept results from observations of the effect of geographic space on therapeutic behavior associated with mental health. The theory has been subjected to test after test against real world data from such places as Denmark, Connecticut, California, Minnesota, Pennsylvania, and Wisconsin and against a substantial number of controls, to the point that, at least within the public health literature, it is referred to as "law." Upon a complete reading of this section, some are certain to be distraught over the title given to the concept. The issue of just what constitutes a "law" in the social sciences including geography has yet to be decided.[1] We present the following as a most interesting case study, which may serve as a prototype for studies in other areas of health care.

Origin

Around the middle of the nineteenth century, the United States, as well as many other "modern" nations, was becoming alarmed over what appeared to be an increasing rate of mental illness among the population—or, as it was stated slightly less delicately at that time, the fact that "to an alarming extent the number of lunatics, when compared with the population, is continually on the increase."[2] Edward Jarvis, was particularly concerned about whether "lunacy" was increasing, stationary, or diminishing, in proportion to the increase in the general population.

He believed that the opening of more insane asylums for the "cure or the protection of lunatics, the spread of their reports, the extension of the knowledge of their character, power, and usefulness by the means of the patients that they protect and cure, have created and continue to create more and more interest in the subject of insanity, and more confidence in its curability."

> [And] consequently, more and more persons and families, who, or such as who, formerly kept their insane friends and relatives at home, or allowed them to stroll abroad about the streets or country, now believe that they can be restored, or improved or at least made more comfortable in these public institutions—thus lists swell of inmates.[3]

Based on the above considerations Jarvis states the following, which is the essence of his "law": *"The people in the vicinity of lunatic hospitals send more patients to them than those at a greater distance."* Thus, preceding Stewart[4] and Zipf[5] by almost a hundred years and Ravenstein[6] by some twenty-three years, Jarvis observed the "inverse distance law" operating among mental patients and proposed that this was related to some decay of information away from the community in which the mental hospital is located. Jarvis' specific statements were in opposition to some observers'. At that time there were substantial differences in the interpretation of the spatial distribution of mental illness. Jarvis included empirical evidence to logically counter these suggestions.

Admission rates of counties containing asylums were compared with distant counties. The county of Worcester, Massachusetts, site of an asylum, "has sent one lunatic out of every 116 of its population, while the most remote counties of the state have sent only one in 361 of their people to the state hospital"; the county of Oneida, New York, "has sent one in 361, and the remotest counties sent only one in 1,523 of their population"; the people of Fayette County, Kentucky, "sent one in 89 of their people to the lunatic hospital, while the farthest counties sent only one in 1,635 of their population." Quoting similar circumstances for a number of other states including Maine, New Hampshire, Ohio, and Maryland, he asked whether "we should infer that the numbers of the insane, in proportion to the whole numbers of the people, was three times as prevalent in Worcester as in Barnstable and Berkshire Counties in Massachusetts; four times as frequent in Oneida as in

Cattaraugus and Chatauque Counties, in New York; and eighteen times as frequent in Fayette as in Macracken and Hickman Counties in Kentucky." Such deductions, he suggests would be manifestly absurd.

Similar findings were demonstrated later for Denmark. In 1879, Selmer observed that the admissions rates from local areas to a state hospital were greater than those to the same hospital from more distant areas.[7] These findings were substantiated later (in 1954) by Svendsen.[8] Nevertheless it appears that Jarvis was the first to observe this phenomenon.

Literature pertaining to this phenomenon is wanting for almost a hundred years after the original observations. Perhaps, at the risk of being facetious, the law was overshadowed by Jarvis' other findings important to the "scientific" study of psychiatry; for instance, "disturbances of the brain" could be caused by sleeping in a barn filled with new hay, by excessive labor, by intemperance in snuff, by excessive study (almost universally supported even today by the majority of our students), by blowing the fife all night, and by preaching the gospel for sixteen days and nights. Probably the correct reasons for the scarcity of studies is that only within the past decade or so has there been a substantial effort directed toward development of mental health programs for both rural and urban areas stressing "local" community involvement. The result has been an increased emphasis on planning for the delivery of mental health services.

In most recommendations of the United States, as well as other countries, there is a plea for more and smaller mental hospitals. The catchment area of each hospital will, as a consequence, be reduced. A most persistent problem is the delineation of the service area that a facility can serve adequately. While there have been guidelines established for the size of the population best served by a full-time mental team of a psychiatrist, a psychologist, and a social worker, there is no suggestion of the optimum geographic area to be served by either the rural or urban mental health facilities.[9]

Each of the following studies tests the null hypothesis that there is no decrease in the number of admissions to a mental hospital with increasing distance of residence from the hospital. The assumption is that with increasing distance of residence from a mental hospital there is a lower probability of admission. The studies selected for this chapter provide a series of interesting attendant and corollary hypotheses, but space is a constraint that will limit our discussion. While the degree of rejection of the hypothesis varies among the studies, it may be stated that each finds Jarvis' Law to be in effect among the sample populations.

Admission rates (average annual number of patients first admitted divided by the population exposed to risk during the specified interval) for the state mental hospital of Wisconsin were examined for a series of concentric zones that were drawn about the county in which the facility is located.[10] The annual rates of first admissions per 100,000 population declined progressively from a high of ninety-eight in the county of the hospital to sixty-two for counties within fifty miles of the facility. Further, the rate was forty-five for counties between fifty and a hundred miles away, and thirty-three for counties over a hundred miles from the hospital. Similar results were observed for admission rates by concentric rings (see Figures 6.1 and 6.2) drawn about the Warren

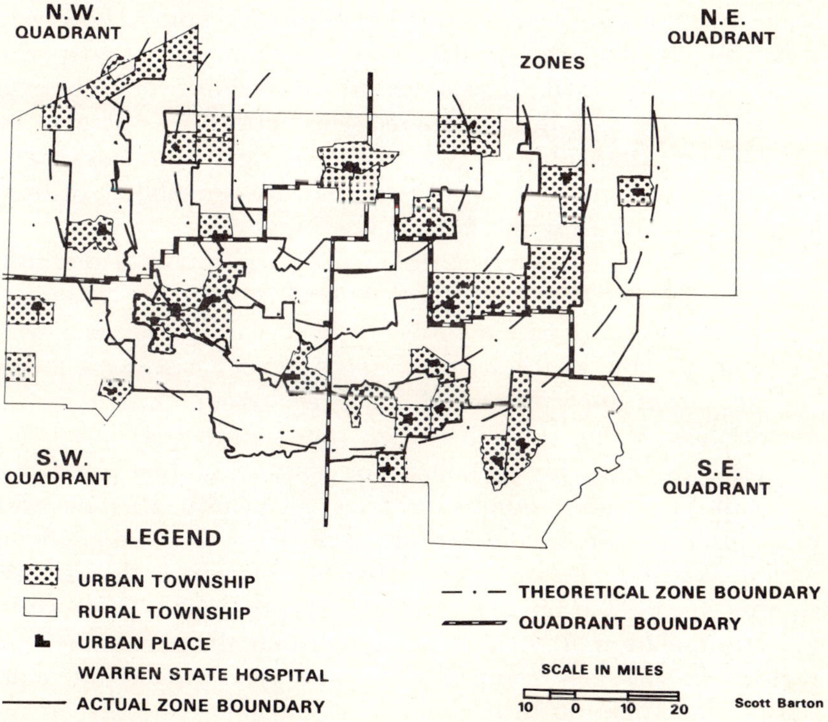

Figure 6.1. Zones, quadrants and type of residential area, Warren State Hospital service area.

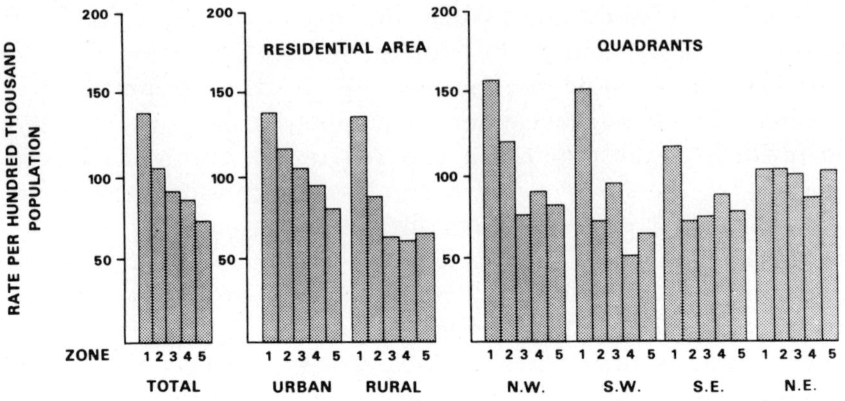

Figure 6.2. Warren State Hospital admission rates per 100,000 population, 1948-52.

State Hospital in Pennsylvania.[11] In this study, however, the area was divided into quadrants and different functional relationships were obtained. The rates of admission were observed to decline in three of the quadrants. The decay was not observed in one (NE) quadrant, but in two (NW, SW) significant linear relationships were present. The hypothesis that the probability of hospitalization is greater near the facility was supported.

The differential effect of distance by age group is presented in Figure 6.3. Briefly, there are several interesting observations: admission rates for patients seventy-five years of age and over are the highest, and all these rates generally decrease with increasing distance from the hospital. In this age group, urban males and females have higher rates than their rural counterparts.

Similar findings are obtained for a study of first admissions in Denmark.[12] First admission rates of nearby Risskov and the most distant town in the district, Aalborg, were compared for the period 1949-51 (Figure 6.4). Table 6.1 illustrates first admissions appears to be particularly greatest for the aged (over sixty-five years) population. It is also interesting that the admission rates for females in the age group 25-44 years were essentially equal in Aarhus and Aalborg. In the remaining categories the first admission rates were higher in the nearer town than in the more distant zone.[13]

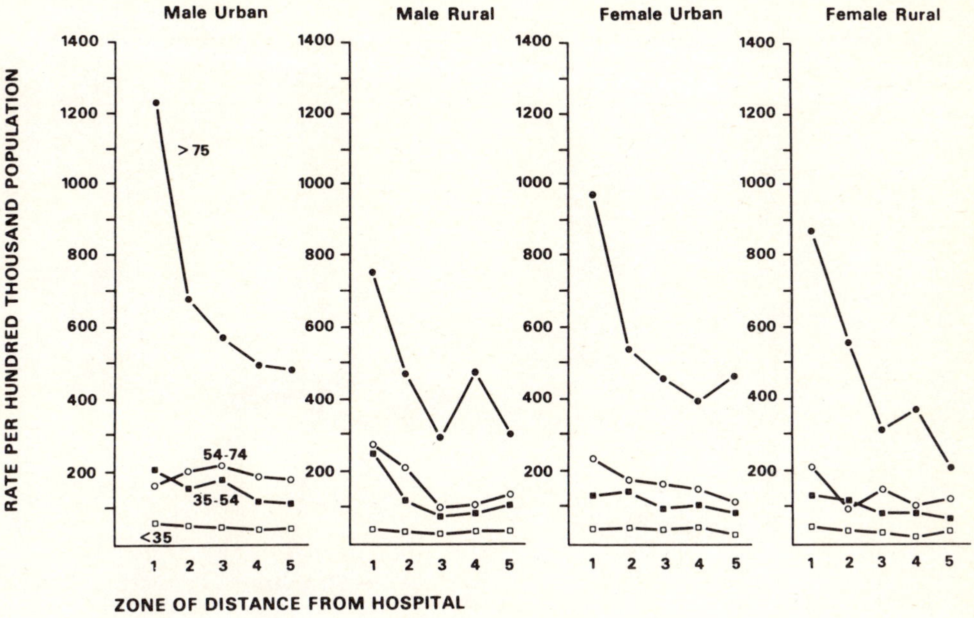

Figure 6.3. Estimated average annual first admission rates per 100,000 population, Warren State Hospital, 1948-52.

Probably the most comprehensive investigations into Jarvis' Law are those by Sohler.[14] Her objective was to "resolve suggestions that Jarvis' Law is an artifact resulting from the chance operation of confounding factors including the distribution of high-risk groups (the elderly, the disadvantaged, or the non-white), the urban-rural continuum and the location of alternative services."[15] Distance zones were constructed centered upon the Connecticut State Hospitals and admission rates per 10,000 population within these zones were examined. The findings are illustrated in Figure 6.5.

For all ages there appears to be an inverse relationship between first admission rate and distance of residence from hospital. For those age groups under sixty-five the admission rates of the inner zones are often double and sometimes triple those of the outermost zones. For the female age groups over sixty-five the slope is very steep, the proximal rate being almost ten times that of the outer zones.

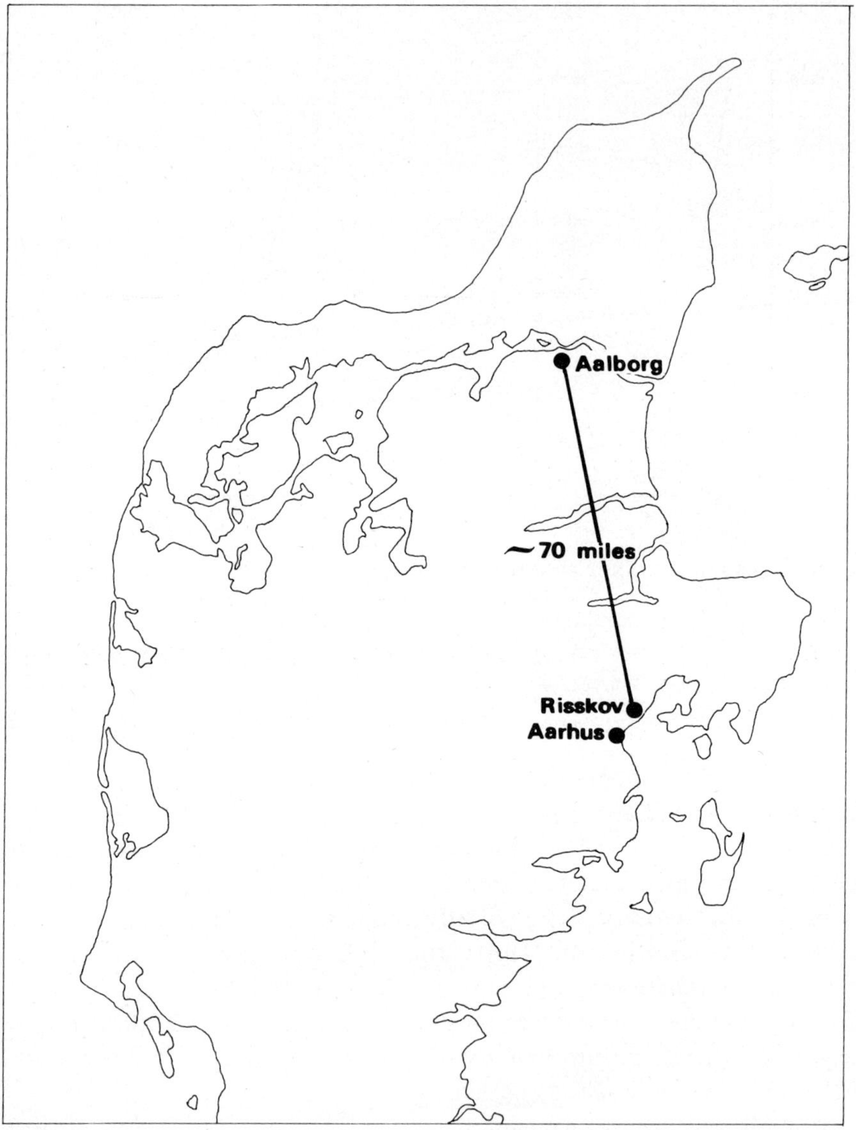

Figure 6.4. Map of Jutland.

Table 6.1. First admission rates to mental hospital from Aarhus and Aalborg

	Rates per 100,000 adult population			
	Male		*Female*	
Age	*Aarhus*	*Aalborg*	*Aarhus*	*Aalborg*
Average	286	142	222	181
15–24	266	122	308	195
25–44	314	175	204	205
45–64	275	140	184	177
65 +	245	37	239	64

Source: M. Bille, 1963.

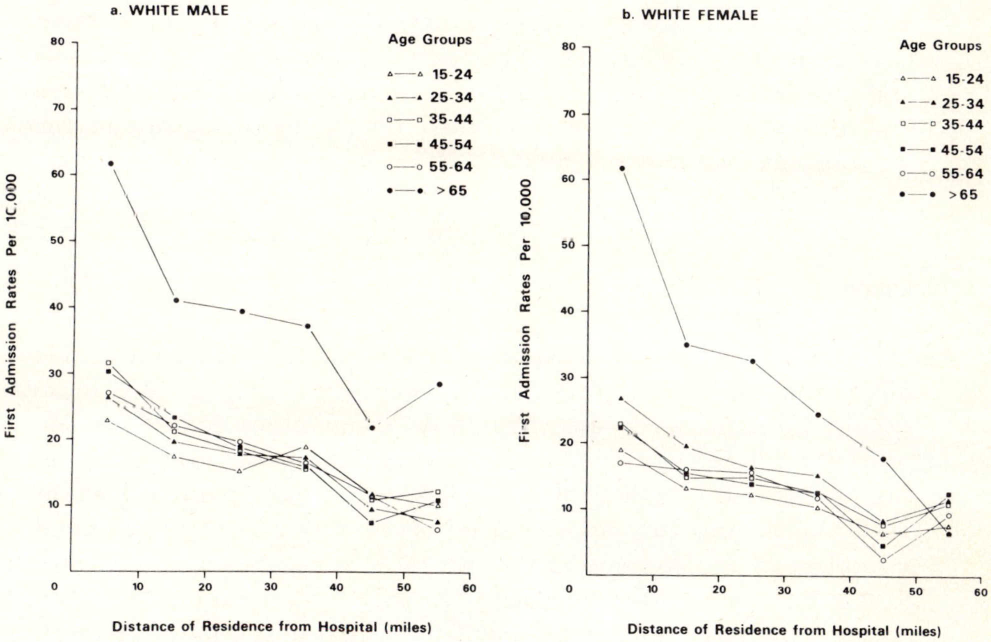

Figure 6.5. Warren State Hospital first admission rates per 10,000 white male and white female.

Controls were then applied to investigate the possibility of the admission rates being an artifact of those factors mentioned above. It was discovered, though differences in decay rates were obtained, that Jarvis' "law" could not be shaken by controls for metropolitan and non-metropolitan areas, high poverty and low poverty towns, white and black populations, and less severe disorders and functional psychoses. For each of the categories examined, the effect was found to be higher in the former group than the latter. Finally, the role of alternative psychiatric services were examined for their influence on admission rates. The conclusions are similar. Jarvis' law does not disappear among towns when controlled by the number of alternative sources of care. It was evident in the group of towns without any service and "clearly perceptible in the groups of towns with limited service." It did not entirely disappear even within the "gravitational field" of the comprehensive service offered in Hartford.

The conclusions from the study are remarkably similar to those of Jarvis, which appeared some hundred years ago. It is suggested that community investment in a new facility is both "the result and the cause of a more hopeful attitude toward psychiatric care and this attitude in turn may be reflected more rapidly in the institution's immediate sphere of influence than in outlying areas."[16]

Diagnostic Differences

Most of the studies investigating Jarvis' Law have demonstrated a differential impact of distance by diagnosis. Most of the more severe disorders, such as schizophrenia and other functional disorders, are least consistent in the relationship between distance and first admission. It is generally concluded that these patients present severe behavioral and emotional problems that cannot be tolerated regardless of the distance to the mental hospital (although evidence does exist that with increasing distance of residence from the hospital the severity of impairment upon first admission is greater). Psychoneurotic patients, usually demonstrating less problematic behavior and attendant social difficulties are most consistently influenced by distance or residence from hospital. It may be that a family might place more value on keeping the patient at home and enduring the consequent difficulties than in placing the patient in the more remote mental hospital.[17] This may be most important in explaining the substantial effect of distance upon the elderly afflicted with diseases of the senium (aging of the brain). When the prognosis is almost certainly death, families more distant from facilities may be more willing to endure hardships associated with the disease in order to keep the family intact. These findings are in complete agreement with the suggested relationships of distance and illness and therapeutic behavior presented earlier. In fact, Person (1962) states that the distance factor may be involved in an individual's willingness to recognize and take action to alleviate his own emotional problems.[18]

Jarvis' Law and Planning for Mental Health Delivery

The promise of Jarvis' law for mental health planning specifically, and all health planning generally, centers primarily upon the potential for estimating facility size necessary to provide health care as well as case load mix, given some predetermined geographical service area. We must also view the mapping of disease incidence rates with skepticism until controlled for the effect of spatial differentials in utilization of health services and treatment of illnesses. The presence of more numerous hospitals and facilities must be associated with a reduction in service-area size. This reduction will tend to eliminate the low rates of admission associated with more distant communities. However, the high proximal rates tend to be increased with this reduction. It has been estimated, for example, that the result of this effort in California would be to double the demand for psychiatric services.[19] In some sections of Connecticut a reduction of service area would result in an estimated eightfold increase in admissions from some zones.[20] Similarly, the differential impact upon various age groups and diagnoses can be estimated for defined areas contributing to a more accurate estimation of both volume and type of services required.

Perhaps the designation "law" attached to the observations of the investigations discussed above is premature. There has been no systematic investigation of the distance decay to determine the stability of various descriptive functions as there has been in the analysis of the gravity formulation by Zipf. The findings, indeed, may be similar for both, namely: "the rate of change in admissions over distance varies over time, according to place, and according to social characteristics in the population."[21] Jarvis' law does provide planners with a potentially effective tool for investigation and (hopefully) future research will contribute to an increased recognition of the associated parameters and their effects.

REFERENCES CITED

[1] D. Harvey, "Laws and Theories in Geography," Chapter 9 in *Explanation in Geography,* St. Martin's Press, New York, 1969.

[2] E. Jarvis, "On the Supposed Increase of Insanity," *The American Journal of Insanity,* vol. VIII, 1851-52, pp. 333-364.

[3] Ibid., p. 334.

[4] J. Q. Stewart, "Demographic Gravitation: Evidence and Applications," *Sociometry,* vol. 11, 1948, pp. 31-56.

[5] G. K. Zipf, *Human Behavior and the Principle of Least Effort,* Cambridge, Massachusetts, 1949.

[6] E. G. Ravenstein, "Laws of Migration," 1885.

[7] H. Selmer, Statistike Meddelser og, Undersogelser fra Sindssygeanstalten ved Aarhus i dens forste 25 Aar 1852-77, Kjobenhavn.

[8] F. B. Svendsen, "Patientskiftea pa sindssygehospitalet ved Aarhus 1952," *Ugekr. Laeg.* 116, pp. 1050-1053.

[9] A. Hodges and H. Dorken, "Location and Outpatient Psychiatric Care," *Public Health Reports,* vol. 76, no. 3, March 1961, pp. 239-241.

[10] B. Weiss, J. R. Macaulay and A. Pincus, "Geographic Location and State Hospital Utilization," *American Journal of Psychiatry,* vol. 124, no. 5, November 1967, pp. 91-95.

[11] P. H. Person, Jr., "Geographic Variation in First Admissions to a State Hospital," *Public Health Reports,* vol. 77, August 1962, pp. 719-731.

[12] M. Bille, "The Influence of Distance on Admissions to Mental Hospitals," *Acta Psychiatrica Scandinavia,* Supplementum, 169, vol. 39, 1963, pp. 226-233.

[13] Ibid., p. 231.

[14] K. B. Sohler and J. D. Thompson, "Jarvis' Law and the Planning of Mental Health Services," *Public Health Reports,* vol. 85, no. 6, June 1970, pp. 503-510, and K. B. Sohler, "The Role of Alternative Psychiatric Service in Connecticut," *Public Health Reports,* vol. 85, no. 6, June 1970, pp. 511-516.

[15] Sohler, p. 503.

[16] Ibid., p. 513.

[17] Person, p. 730.

[18] Ibid.

[19] M. S. Blumberg, "Psychiatric Bed Needs: Factors Relating to Demand for Psychiatric Services in California," California Department of Mental Hygiene, Sacramento, August 1965.

[20] Sohler and Thompson, op. cit., p. 508.

[21] T. Hagerstrand, "Migration and Area," in *Migration in Sweden—A Symposium, ed. by D. Hannerberg, T. Hagerstrand and B. Odeving, Lund* Studies in Geography, Series B, no. 13, 1957, in Harvey, 1969.

Chapter VII

IMPACT OF GEOGRAPHIC FACTORS ON HEALTH CARE:

The Provider

In the two previous chapters our attention focused primarily upon the impact of geographic and associated factors as they affect patient utilization of health services. Of course, the provider is of equal importance. The literature pertaining to the effect of these factors on the providers of care is certainly not as extensive as that relating to the client. The results, however, are extremely interesting and potentially significant and most important to the planning and delivery of health care. Evidence of the impact of geographic factors is presented below as it pertains to the physician's utilization of hospital services, and physicians.

We have witnessed within the United States an increasing sophistication of medical technology to the extent that the normal practice of medicine is rarely carried on in isolation; in fact, most physicians have contact or appointments with hospitals. (This reason is most commonly cited for the decrease in home visits by physicians.) A study conducted in North Carolina examined the relationship between the physician and the hospital.[1] The major thrust of this study was to isolate factors that determine how actively each physician exercised hospital privileges either for the purpose of patient care or for improving his own professional skills.[2] Of those variables considered, it appears that distance represents a major reason for the lack of active participation and utilization of available services. A summary table (Table 7.1) indicating a moderate decay of physicians utilization of hospital services is presented below. The percentage of doctors actively using the hospital declined from a ninety percent level for those with practices less than six miles from the hospital to a low of forty-two percent for those practicing over fifteen miles away. As might be expected, a substantial number of "inactive" physicians were located in small towns (under 1,000), reflecting the concentration of hospitals in the larger urban areas. In our earlier discussions of physician location, it was observed that these physicians are generally older and have generally less contact, and hence less familiarity, with hospital services. We might, therefore, assume this to be true of the "inactive" physicians. However, there was a statistically significant difference in neither the ages nor training of the "active" and "inactive" physicians. The explanation is apparently not complex; a distance threshold exists (in this case approximately fifteen miles) beyond which the amount of time and effort required to travel for hospital facilities and services in unacceptable. Thus, it is evident that physicians' utilization rates are also affected in a manner similar to those of patients.

Table 7.1. Relationship between distance from hospital and use of hospital

Distance from Nearest Hospital	*Total No. of Doctors*	*No. Who Actively use Hospital*	*Per Cent*
Under 6 miles	62	56	90
6–10 miles	9	7	78
11–15 miles	11	9	82
Over 15 miles	12	5	42

Source: Peterson, et. al., "The Doctor and the Medical Community," *Journal of Medical Education*, vol. 31, December 1956, p. 95.

The Impact of Referral Practices

In the study cited above it was mentioned, almost in passing, that one of the most frequent reasons for selection of consultants was proximity. The conclusions of two subsequent investigations corroborate and emphasize this important relationship.

A report from North Carolina examined the process by which patients are referred to a major university hospital.[3] Physicians' reasons for referral of patients to a medical center were grouped under three headings: (1) referrals initiated by the physician for specific reasons, (2) referrals initiated by the physician for nonspecific reasons, and (3) referrals initiated primarily by the patient (dissatisfaction with physician or economic reasons). For Group 1 it was determined that the referring physician had delineated a patient's problem and had a specific purpose for seeking consultation. Referral resulted from realized limits of practice, insufficient capabilities of the local facilities, or the recognition of an interesting teaching problem. Referrals from Group 2 included such nonspecific reasons as "help in diagnosis and treatment" or "a complete check-up."

Several hypotheses were treated. For instance, the farther a patient has to travel to the medical center, the more specific will be the physician's reason for referral, that is, more specific referrals would be expected (Group 1) from physicians at greater distances from the medical center. Conversely, it would be expected that more patients from nearby areas would be nonspecific (Group 2) or patient-initiated referrals (Group 3). The distance categories utilized are crude; however, the observed results are in the expected direction (Table 7.2).

Seventy-two percent of those patients referred for specific reasons were from distances of at least seventy miles, and only forty-eight percent of the referrals were initiated by patients beyond seventy miles. The percentages are almost inverted in order of magnitude for referrals by physicians whose practices are less than seventy miles from the medical center (Group 1, twenty-eight, Group 2, fifty-two, and Group 3, sixty-five percent respectively). In this instance, there was a difference of seven years in the average age of physicians referring for specific and nonspecific reasons (thirty-eight and forty-five years of age respectively). The

Table 7.2. Reason for referral to medical center by distance of practice from medical center

Reason Group	Less than 70 miles		70 miles and Over		All Groups	
	No.	%	No.	%	No.	%
1. Physician-initiated referrals for specific reason	5	28	13	72	18	100
2. Physician-initiated referrals for non-specific reasons	12	52	11	48	23	100
3. Referrals initiated primarily by patients	28	65	15	35	43	100
Totals	45	54*	39	46	46	100

Source: Williams, et. al., "Patient Referral to a University Clinic: Patterns in a Rural State," *American Journal of Public Health*, vol. 50, no. 10, p. 1503.

distance factor again emerges as an "operator" in the provision of health delivery, although apparently unrecognized by the physicians themselves.[4]

From England, more specifically the Oxford Record Linkage Study (O.R.L.S.) area, comes our final and perhaps most significant contribution that relates geographic factors to physician referral practices.[5] The study is examined in some detail due to the perceived importance.

Perinatal mortality experienced in the Oxford area in 1962 is examined as it relates to several variables. Of significant interest, is the relationship between perinatal mortality and the variation in the use of consultant obstetric services by general practitioners. Moreover, the factors that influence this behaivor are investigated.

The organization of obstetric services for the area include (1) consultant groups at a teaching hospital, (2) a combined consultant and general practitioner (G.P.) unit as a district hospital, and (3) three G.P. units. General practitioner units differ from consultant units in the former's lack of a resident medical officer and blood bank. Operating and anaesthetic facilities limit practice to the application of forceps or the use of surgical induction procedures and render caesarean sections out of the question. G.P. units, do offer advantages over delivery at home. They have a trained midwife who is always immediately available. Further, the presence of labor rooms and the accessibility to emergency ambulance services offer other advantages. These units are generally located in small towns from six to twelve miles from the nearest consultant unit.[6]

Within this framework of health delivery the study investigated 5300 births of mothers who were classified into three risk groups:

Group I (high risk): all mothers over the age of thirty-five years, nulliparae over thirty, multiparae (having had four or more children) and mothers with a past history of still birth

Group II (intermediate risk): all nulliparae not included in the above

Group III (low risk): all other mothers

As expected from the high ratio of high-risk mothers in Group I, perinatal mortality rates for consultant units are slightly (not statistically significantly) higher than for deliveries at home and at the G.P. units.

Fifty-five practices selected for study were divided into two groups according to the presence or absence of accessible G.P. unit beds. Practices were classified as having access to G.P. units when the distance to such a unit was less than that to the nearest consultant unit.[7] Further, each of these two main groups of practices were subdivided according to the distance between the office and the nearest consultant unit. This classification was based on travelling time by public transport from each practice to the nearest consultant unit. The tendency to "book" or refer patients by travelling time to the nearest consultant unit for practices with and without access to G.P. units is presented below in Table 7.3.

This table shows that when G.P. beds are most accessible the effect of distance on the percentage of mothers referred for consultant care decreased with increasing distance from the consulting unit.

Similarities between patient and physician behavior may be illustrated by the conclusion drawn by Weiss, et. al. for travel patterns to

Table 7.3. Proportion of cases referred and the perinatal mortality rate by travelling time to the nearest consultant unit for practices with and without access to G. P. units.

	Practices with Access to G. P. Units				*Practices w/o Access to G. P. Units*			
Travelling-time to Consultant Unit	*No. of Practices*	*No. of Cases*	*Cases Referred for Consultant Care*	*Perinatal Mortality rate/1000*	*No. of Practices*	*No. of Cases*	*Cases Referred for Consultant Care*	*Perinatal Mortality rate/1000*
0–20 minutes	4	537	42%	20	25	2,057	60%	18
21–40 minutes	8	1,078	27%	28	6	693	49%	22
Over 40 minutes	5	293	9%	44	7	530	52%	21
Total	17	1,908	28%	28	38	3,280	53%	19

Source: Hobbs and Acheson, 1966, p. 502. Table IV.

> clinics of group practice members in Seattle.[8] That "a larger proportion of patients will use the nearest clinic when the nearest clinic is relatively close and the distance to the alternative clinic is great. But, when the distance both to the nearest and to the more distant clinics is absolutely greater, but the clinics are almost equally distant from the patient's residence, the proportion of visits to the alternative clinics increases."[9]

When G.P. units are not accessible the effect of distance on referral to consultants is substantially reduced. Most importantly, there is a significant trend for perinatal mortality to increase in association with the decreasing percentage of cases booked at consultant units. The total percentage (twenty-eight percent) of mothers booked for consultant care when G.P. units are accessible is substantially less than the percentage (fifty-three percent) booked for consultant care when G.P. units are not available. Again, the perinatal mortality in the practices with access to G.P. units (twenty-eight per 1000) is significantly higher than in the practices without access to G.P. units (nineteen per 1000).[10]

It is further observed that when G.P. beds are available, referrals to consultant units decline sharply as distance increases, regardless of the risk group of the mother. This becomes extremely important for high-risk mothers (Group I). For practices where G.P. beds are most accessible, the percentages of high-risk mothers referred for specialist care by distance intervals of zero to twenty, twenty-one to forty, and over forty minutes from the nearest consultant unit are fifty-three percent, thirty-eight percent, and twelve percent respectively. When G.P. beds are available locally, distance has a profound effect on the referral patterns of all risk groups of mothers for consultant care.[11] The perinatal mortality in Group I (mothers referred from practices with access to G.P. units) is forty-seven per 1,000, while that for the remaining practices is only nineteen per 1,000—a significant difference. Significant differences were also observed among Group II mothers. (Again there are no significant differences in the socio-economic status, etc., of the mothers.)

It may be generally concluded that a "convenience factor" associated with functional geographic space is operating in the obstetric referral patterns of physicians. It may also be concluded that as a result, many mothers are referred to inappropriate facilities. While less important to low-risk mothers, this "improper" behavior on the part of the physician is responsible for a significantly higher perinatal mortality rate among high-risk mothers. These observed relationships establish a link between referral patterns, the spatial distribution of health facilities, and life itself.

REFERENCES CITED

[1] O. L. Peterson, L. P. Andrews, R. S. Spain and B. G. Greenberg, "An Analytical Study of North Carolina General Practice, 1953-1954," *Journal of Medical Education,* vol. 31, December 1956, pp. 94-103.
[2] Ibid., p. 94.
[3] T. F. Williams, K. S. White, L. P. Andrews, E. Diamond, B. G. Greenberg, A. A. Hammrick and E. A. Hunter, "Patient Referral to a University Clinic: Patterns in a Rural State," *American Journal of Public Health,* vol. 50, no. 10, 1960, pp. 1493-1507.
[4] Williams, et al., pp. 1503-1504.
[5] M. S. T. Hobbs and E. D. Acheson, "Perinatal Mortality and the Organization of Obstetric Services in the Oxford Area in 1962," *British Medical Journal,* February 26, 1966, pp. 499-505.
[6] Ibid., p. 499.
[7] Ibid., p. 502.
[8] J. E. Weiss, M. M. Greenlick and J. F. Jones, "Determinants of Medical Care Utilization: The Impact of Spatial Factors," *Inquiry,* vol. VIII, no. 4, pp. 50-57.
[9] Ibid., p. 55.
[10] Hobbs, op. cit., p. 502.
[11] Ibid., p. 502.

Chapter VIII

IMPACT OF GEOGRAPHIC FACTORS ON INSTITUTIONAL POLICIES

Geographic factors have been identified as important and "valid" influences on utilization rates of hospitals by physicians and their referral practices. In this chapter we present initial evidence suggesting that geographic factors may also be influential in the length of hospital stay, the actual modes of treatment, and diffusion of innovative health plans.

Several hypotheses were examined relating spatial factors to the release of patients from state mental hospitals in Wisconsin.[1] The hypotheses suggest that the length of hospital stay varies directly with the distance of a patient's home community from the hospital and, further, that the type of release, as well as the degree of impairment upon release, will vary with the same distance.

Service areas around each state hospital were divided into four distance zones. Zone 1, the county in which the hospital is located; Zone 2, those counties within fifty miles of the hospital facility; Zone 3, counties between fifty and a hundred miles of the hospital; and Zone 4, counties over a hundred miles away. (Patients may come from as far as 280 miles.) Observations on the impact of geographic distance of residence from hospitals on length of stay are provided in Table 8.1, which indicates the distance impact on the type of release from the hospital. It should be mentioned that all findings reported in these tables are valid when controls involving diagnosis, type of admission, level of impairment on admission, sex, type of treatment, and living arrangements on admission or release are applied.[2]

Table 8.1. Duration of stay for all patients and type of release by physicians

Duration of Stay	*Zone 1* *n = 169*	*Zone 2* *n = 282*	*Zone 3* *n = 205*	*Zone 4* *n = 213*
		(in percent)		
0–2 months	63	51	44	37
2–6 months	25	32	34	35
Over 6 months	12	17	22	28

Type of Release	*Zone 1* *n = 99*	*Zone 2* *n = 127*	*Zone 3* *n = 67*	*Zone 4* *n = 93*
Direct Discharge	65	56	28	28
Conditional Release	35	44	72	72

Source: Weiss, et. al., p. 410.

The geographic distance of residence from the mental hospital is significantly associated with the likelihood of release. For both early release (under two months) and stays of longer than six months, patients from nearer the hospital are more likely to be released than those from more distant communities. Similarly, the probability of remaining longer in a hospital increases with increasing distance of residence from the facility. Comparable results have been obtained for London, England, by Norris.[3] Of further interest is the fact that the chances of obtaining an unconditional or direct discharge also decrease with increasing distance. Those patients discharged residing in Zone 1 were also found to be rated more severly impaired when compared to those discharged living in Zones 2 through 4 and the proportion of discharged patients who received chemotherapy was significantly greater with increasing distance of residence from the hospital.

These findings suggest (in addition to the rather pragmatic observation of some of our more astute students that one should always, upon admittance, have in mind a nearby address) that the geographic factor may be one more determining factor contributing to the increasing realization that the hospital careers of mental patients are not entirely determined by their clinical condition.[4] Both release policies and type of treatment appear to be affected.

Spatial Diffusion of Innovative Health Care Plans

Spatial components of institutional and program policies may also contribute to the success or failure of attempts to reorganize health care delivery and provide alternative modes of delivery. This has been particularly demonstrated for the spatial diffusion of acceptance of prepaid group practice plans.

Comprehensive medical care at reasonable cost is desirable for all people. An important step was taken within the United States to initiate group practice prepayment plans that purport to provide comprehensive and continuous medical care service with substantial savings to the consumer. An apparent discrepancy exists, however, between the slow growth of these plans and the general advocacy of group practice prepayment by students of medical care.[5] The study of this discrepancy has many facets. From the social science standpoint this encompasses such important areas of social dynamics as innovation adoption, behavioral aspects of choice and decision, and social influence and communication.[6] Researchers have investigated various socio-psychological factors that relate to the choice of health care plans in situations of dual choice.* Distinct from but related to, the various factors involving the acceptance of group practice is the observable fact of a completed process that is spatially distributed.

*The concept of "dual choice" is used in various places in the U.S. in which prepaid group is offered on a choice basis with the Blue Cross and Blue Shield as the usual alternative. This arrangement of dual choice has been promoted by labor unions.

Sociological investigation of the diffusion of innovations has traditionally been non-geographic in nature, focusing on the decision-making process and the channels and controls exerted on this process by various social structures.[7] From a geographic point of view, acceptance patterns can be described both temporally and spatially. In addition, there are apparently dicisions made by those offering various alternative forms of health care, either explicit or implicit in the organizational framework, that operate to limit the spatial diffusion of acceptance.

Previous work by Metzner and Bashshur indicate some of the difficulties involved in establishing predictive models concerning the acceptance of medical care plans. Among them, the distance factor has been acknowledged as substantial. They suggest that "a satisfactory way of disentangling distance from other variables and measuring the importance of distance has not been achieved."[8]

Distance and associated factors have been identified as significant factors related to the utilization of health resources outside the auspices of certain plans.[9] Distance has also been acknowledged as a significant factor in the initial choice to enroll in a prepaid group practice plan within the dual choice option. Bashshur and Metzner find that residential distance from the affiliated hospital appears to substantially affect enrollment behavior.[10] They found that the acceptance rate in postal zones nearest the only affiliated hospital to be almost twice the rate of acceptance for more distant zones. The nodal characteristic of the acceptance rate demonstrated in Figure 8.1 (a, b, and c) is reinforced by an administrative decision to limit the physician home call area to that illustrated in Figure 8.2. It would appear that diffusion of acceptance of the plan is restrained by both the general impact of geographic space or "friction of distance" generally associated with client behavior and an explicit policy statement by the providers of the health care plan. A somewhat successful attempt has been made to replicate this spatial diffusion pattern using Hagerstrand's Monte Carlo spatial simulation model.[11]

Spatial Interaction and Hospital Services Areas

The study of Ciocco and Altman, discussed earlier, was significant in being among the first attempts to establish a quantitative index

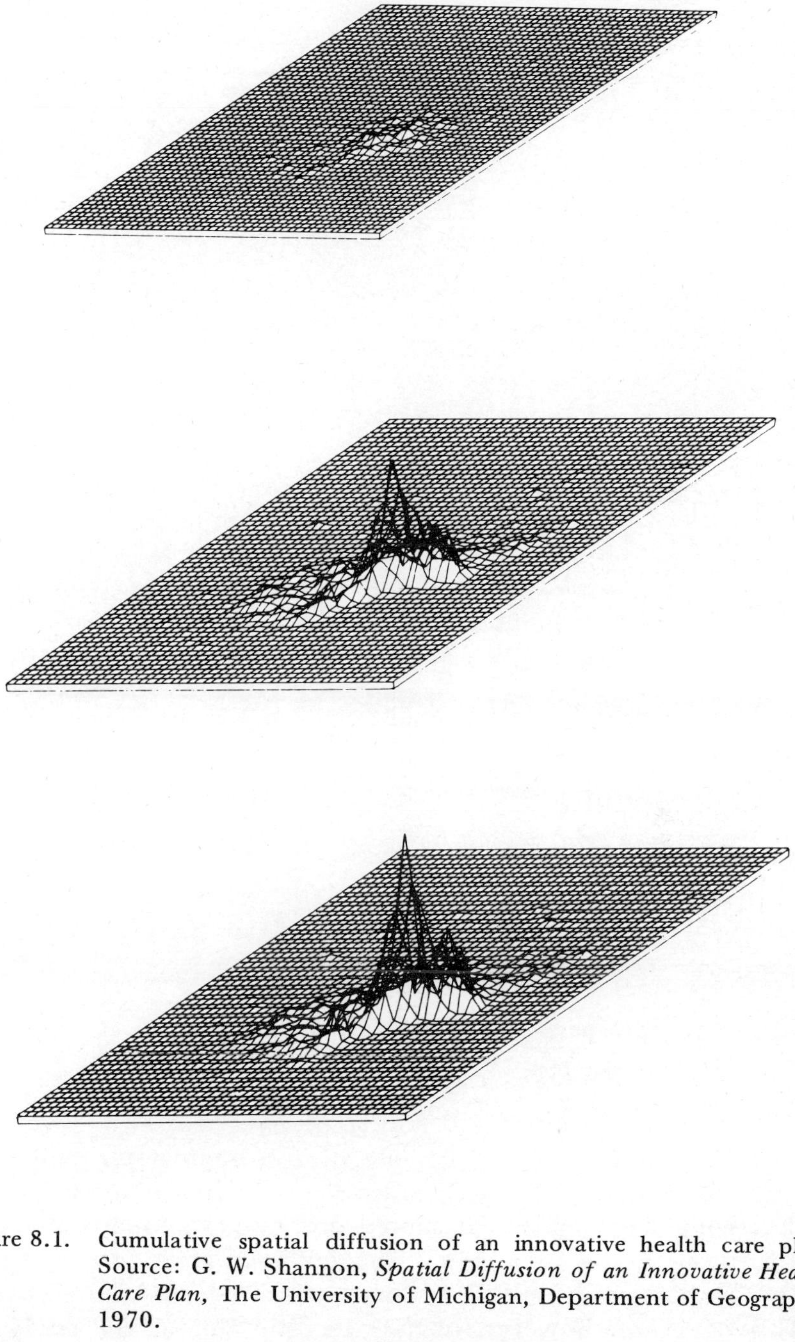

Figure 8.1. Cumulative spatial diffusion of an innovative health care plan. Source: G. W. Shannon, *Spatial Diffusion of an Innovative Health Care Plan*, The University of Michigan, Department of Geography, 1970.

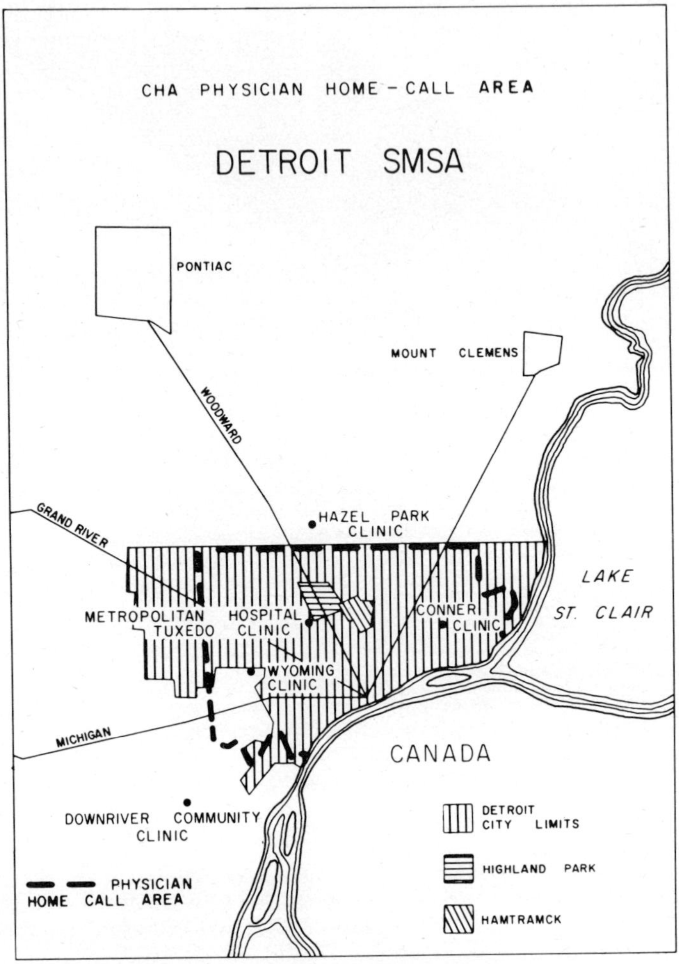

Figure 8.2. CHA physician home-call area, Detroit SMSA.

of "medical service areas" and in the sophistication with which distance was analyzed. Part one of the monograph explores the "use of several statistical indexes as a first approach toward developing some objective, simple, and rapid method of delineating a medical service area."[12] The methods and indexes suggested by Ciocco and Altman have been criticized by later researchers. This does not, however, obviate recognition of the study as an important step in investigating medical service areas. Among their conclusions, Ciocco and Altman emphasized that medical services available in an area should be measured in relation to the actual population served and that knowledge of the pattern of movement from medical care is a prerequisite to the delineation of medical service areas. Their definition of medical service, or "catchment," area expressed the concept of self-containment reproduced in a later U.S. Public Health Service recommendation that this area be:

> The geographic territory from which patients come or are expected to come to existing or proposed hospital or medical facilities, the delineation of which is based on such factors as population distribution, natural geographic boundaries, and transportation and trade patterns, and all parts of which are reasonably accessible to existing or proposed hospital or medical facilities.[13]

This definition represents a substantial improvement over the arbitrary limits suggested earlier—that the jurisdiction of a local health unit "should be limited to a maximum area of 10,000 square miles and that the diameter of the unit should be no more than 100 miles," a measure that apparently disregards a concomitant requirement that the population served be at least 35,000.[14]

Such "rule-of-thumb" limits to travel were applied in an attempt to regionalize rural health care for an economically depressed area of northern Michigan (Figure 8.3). Little Traverse Hospital at Petoskey was selected as the regional hospital for both St. Ignace and Onaway because it was equidistance from the two small communities. Articles of agreement were drawn up between the local health centers and the hospital in 1952. Suffice it to say, the program met with little success. Among the problems ultimately responsible was the lack of enthusiasm on the part of health center staff and local citizenry, particularly those of St. Ignace. Upon reflection, this is not surprising. In calculating the distance separating the local community from the regional hospital, those offering "professional guidance and financial assistance" neglected to consider that for the first five years of the program the forty miles included the unspanned Straits of Mackinac, St. Ignace being in the northern and Petoskey in the southern peninsula of Michigan. Until the completion of a connecting bridge in 1957 the primary connection involved the use of an automobile ferry. From personal experiences, aside from the fare of approximately $5.00, crossing "expenses" could include, at one time or another, any one of

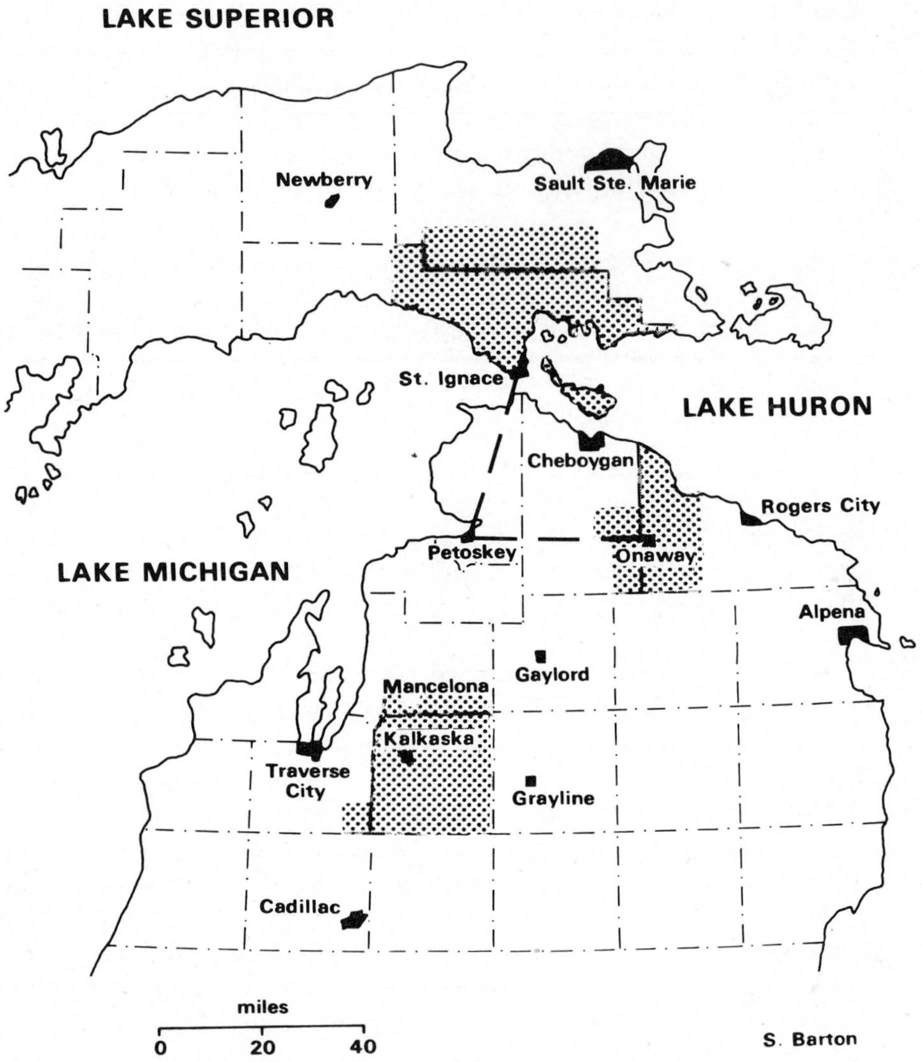

Figure 8.3. Regionalization of health care in northern Michigan. Source: W. J. McNerney and D. C. Riedel, *Regionalization and Rural Health Care*, The University of Michigan, Ann Arbor, 1962.

various combinations of the following: a minimum of one hour wating time to drive onto the ferry and approximately the same amount of time to drive off (In the height of the tourist season,

June through September, and hunting season the wait for boarding could extend well beyond 5 hours); bad-weather crossings (difficult even for the healthy); and days when, of course, crossings were impossible. The use of a functional distance including transportation mode and time, was not employed by those health planners.[15]

The role of transportation networks in the demand for a utilization of medical services also relates to the analysis of "optimal" location of health facilities. The notion of highway impact has been intuitively applied in research on construction of satellite hospitals.[16] Use of transportation and travel time information in hospital and health facility planning was suggested by the American Hospital Association and the Public Health Service in a joint 1961 report.[17]

Time criteria have been established as measures of accessibility in Cincinnati[18] and by the California Department of Public Health.[19] Moreover, a study by Lubin and associates utilized travel-time distance reflecting the value of such information to health facility planning. Attempts at utilizing travel-time intervals in the delineation of meaningful hospital service areas on a patient-distribution basis and on the basis of distance between hospitals have been fruitful.[20] Analysis of total costs, including the size, organizational, and travel components clearly indicates the importance of understanding these variables in planning. Travel-time increases if more efficient, larger, and fewer, hospitals are built; however, total cost becomes a complicated function.[21] Using either time or distance as a measure of separation has interesting implications for planning. It has been demonstrated, for example, that using linear mileage as a measure of accessibility to medical services implies that the suburban residents are at a "disadvantage." On the other hand, the use of time as a measure of distance, suggests that central city residents travel "further" for care than their suburban counterparts.[22]

The appropriate delineation of medical service areas has received much attention with, as yet, little agreement as to the correct methodology. While an extensive discussion of this aspect of health care delivery is beyond the scope of the present book a brief summary statement is appropriate.

Although many studies have been undertaken to examine the hospital service area, research indicates that a large element of chance—that is, factors unrelated to quality of the system—still exists in the selection of a location for medical facilities. Availability of land at a separate location, legislative interpretation, and the gift of a suitable building have been found to be reasons for relocating hospitals.[23] The element of chance in location may be due, in part, to a yet unsuccessful method of delineating medical service areas and their degree of overlap; and a general lack of knowledge concerning the nature of the spatial context within which the general population operates to obtain medical care. This is apparent in the continuing search for accurate methods of delineating hospital service areas[24] and in attempts at measuring the locational efficiency of the present hospital distributions.[25]

REFERENCES CITED

[1] P. Weiss, J. Macaulay and A. Pincus, "Geographic Factors and the Release of Patients from State Mental Hospitals," *American Journal of Psychiatry*, vol. 123, no. 4, October 1966, pp. 408-412.
[2] Ibid., p. 410.
[3] V. Norris, *Mental Health in London*, 1959.
[4] Weiss et. al., op. cit., p. 408.
[5] C. A. Metzner and R. L. Bashshur, "Factors Associated with Choice of Health Care Plan," *Journal of Health and Human Behavior*, vol. 8, no. 4, December 1967, p. 291.
[6] Ibid., p. 291.
[7] E. M. Rogers, *Diffusion of Innovations*, Free Press, New York, 1962.
[8] Metzner and Bashshur, op. cit., p. 291.
[9] E. Friedson, *Patients View of Medical Practice*, Russell Sage Foundation, New York, 1961.
[10] R. L. Bashshur and C. A. Metzner, "Patterns of Social Differentiation Between Community Health Association and Blue Cross-Blue Shield," *Inquiry*, vol. 4, June 1967, pp. 23-44.
[11] G. Shannon, *Spatial Diffusion of an Innovative Health Care Plan*, Michigan Geography Publication No. 3, Department of Geography, University of Michigan, Ann Arbor, 1970, 166 pages.
[12] A. Ciocco and I. Altman, "Medical Service Areas and Distrances Travelled for Physician Care in Western Pennsylvania," *U.S. Public Health Service, Pulbic Health Monograph No. 19*, 1954.
[13] U.S. Department of Health, Education, and Welfare, Public Health Services, *Procedures for Area Health Facility Planning: A Guide for Planning Agencies*, Public Health Science Publications, No. 930-B-3, U.S. Government Printing Office, Washington, D.C., September 1963, p. 118.
[14] J. W. Mountin and C. J. Greve, *Public Health Areas and Hospital Facilities: A Plan for Coordination*, Public Health Service Publication No. 42, U.S. Government Printing Office, Washington, D.C., 1950, p. 4.
[15] W. J. McNerney and D. C. Riedel, *Regionalization and Rural Health Care*, The University of Michigan, Ann Arbor, 1962, p. 209.

[16] C. M. Platuo and D. C. Wegmiller, "Satellite Hospitals to Rise Along Houston's Freeways," *Hospitals,* vol. 37, Part I, August 1, 1963.
W. W. Turner, "Fairview Hospital in Minneapolis Prepares to Start Its First Branch in the Suburbs," *Modern Hospital,* vol. 99, November 1962, p. 94.
W. W. Turner, "Satellite Hospitals Bring Health Care to Suburbanites," *Modern Hospital,* vol. 99, November 1962, p. 92.
P. B. Hallen, "Hospitals Branch-Out: A Study of Multiple-Unit Operations, Part II," *Hospitals,* vol. 37, no. 16, August 16, 1963.

[17] U.S. Public Health Service, "Areawide Planning for Hospitals and Related Health Facilities," PHS Publication No. 855, U.S. Government Printing Office, Washington, D.C., July 1961, p. 28.

[18] Ralph Marrison, "Hospital Service: Time Replaces Space," *Hospitals,* vol. 38, January 16, 1964.

[19] State of California, Department of Public Health: *Hospitals,* Berkeley, August 1964, p. 15.

[20] M. F. Long and P. V. Feldstein, "Economics of Hospital Systems: Peak Loads and Regional Coordination," *American Economic Review,* vol. LVII, May 1967, pp. 119-129.

[21] J. B. Schneider, "Measuring the Locational Efficiency of the Urban Hospital," *Health Services Research,* Summer 1967, pp. 154-169.

[22] G. W. Shannon, J. L. Skinner and R. L. Bashshur, "Time and Distance: The Journey for Health Care," *International Journal of Heatlh Services,* Spring, 1973, pp. 237-244.

[23] P. B. Hallen, "Hospitals Branch-Out: A Study of Multiple-Unit Operations, Part I," *Hospitals,* vol. 37, no. 15, August 1, 1963.

[24] H. D. Cherniack and J. B. Schneider, "A New Approach to the Delineation of Hospital Service Areas," *Discussion Paper Series No. 16,* Regional Science Research Institute, Seattle, Washington, August 1967.
P. F. Gross, "Urban Health Disorders, Spatial Analysis, and the Economics of Health Facility Location," *International Journal of Health Services,* vol. 2, no. 1, February 1972, pp. 63-84.
J. B. Schneider and J. G. Symons, "Regional Health Facility System Planning: An Access Opportunity Approach," Discussion Paper No. 48, Philadelphia, Regional Science Research Institute, 1971.

[25] Schneider, "Measuring the Locational Efficiency of the Urban Hospital," p. 154-169.
R. L. Morrill and M. G. Kelley, "The Simulation of Hospital Use and the Estimation of Location Efficiency," *Geographical Analysis,* vol. II, no. 3, July 1970, pp. 283-300.

Chapter IX

"IF WISHES WERE HORSES . . ."

Health care is a fundamental human right. The problem is one of ensuring this right. The fulfillment of this belief is embodied in numerous and diverse international health care systems. The United States, however, stands alone as the only developed country that has not yet attempted to deliver health care equitably. It is apparent in the uneven distribution and accessibility of health resources (facilities and services) when compared with other modern countries. Attempts to determine parameters associated with physician location are inconclusive and have little utility in light of the current laissez-fare attitude toward the delivery of medicine and the present framework of non-committment to a philosophy of health as a human right. Adam Smith's "invisible hand" is not operating to redress problems related to health delivery.

The health seeker within the United States suffers an inordinate imposition through the development and evolution of distance barriers and conduits, both social and economic as well as geographic. These have been demonstrated to be crucial and detrimental to human health and, ultimately, to life itself. Provider-referral patterns and institutional policies, as they relate to length of stay and mode of treatment, also have demonstrated spatial elements.

Suggestions derived from spatial analysis of the multi-faceted health delivery problem can be and have been recommended here to increase the effectiveness of health care delivery. For instance, increasing accessibility could be obtained through organization of health services along the spatial and functional constructs suggested by central place theory. Further, the behavior by the health seeker and provider as influenced by spatial factors must be included in any comprehensive health care plan. Certain demonstrated institutional policies reflect the need for extended inquiries into patients' rights.

The ultimate recommendation, of course, is a basic committment to a national policy of health care embodying the philosophy that health care is a human right. Failure of the acceptance of such a national policy does not preclude, however, the applicability of spatial/functional investigation and organization at regional and other levels for selected groups.

". . .then beggars would ride." (Mother Goose)